636.08
LEE
11/91

Lee, Mary Price.

Opportunities in
animal and pet care
careers.

$12.95

DATE			

OPPORTUNITIES IN
ANIMAL AND PET
CARE CAREERS

Mary Price Lee
Richard S. Lee

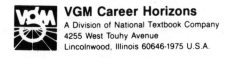

VGM Career Horizons
A Division of National Textbook Company
4255 West Touhy Avenue
Lincolnwood, Illinois 60646-1975 U.S.A.

Photo Credits

Front cover: upper left, American Animal Hospital Association; Davis Animal Hospital, Elkhart, IN; upper right, Zoological Society of Philadelphia; lower left, Zoological Society of Philadelphia; lower right, Smithsonian Institution, National Zoological Park.

Back cover: upper left, Pennsylvania SPCA; upper right, Pennsylvania SPCA; lower left, American Animal Hospital Association; lower right, Smithsonian Institution, National Zoological Park.

1989 Printing

Copyright © 1984 by National Textbook Company
4255 West Touhy Avenue
Lincolnwood (Chicago), Illinois 60646-1975 U.S.A.
All rights reserved. No part of this book may
be reproduced, stored in a retrieval system, or
transmitted in any form or by any means, electronic,
mechanical, photocopying, recording or otherwise,
without the prior permission of National Textbook Company.
Manufactured in the United States of America.
Library of Congress Catalog Number: 84-60168

8 9 0 ML 9 8 7 6 5

ABOUT THE AUTHORS

Mary Price Lee holds an A.B. in English and an M.A. in Education from the University of Pennsylvania. She has published numerous newspaper and magazine articles plus seven nonfiction books for junior high and high school readers. Four of these are career-oriented: *Ms. Veterinarian,* Westminster Press, 1976; *The Team That Runs Your Hospital,* Westminster Press, 1980; *A Career in Pediatrics,* Julian Messner Div. of Simon & Schuster, 1982; and *Your Future in Industrial Research & Development,* Richards Rosen Press, 1983. She is an assiduous researcher, enthusiastic traveler and experienced interviewer.

Richard S. Lee holds an A.B. in English from the College of William and Mary. He has spent his working life in the creative side of advertising, as a copywriter, interviewer/photographer, promotion program coordinator, and currently as an agency creative director. He has written numerous articles and reviews.

This book is the Lees' first collaboration.

ACKNOWLEDGEMENTS

Our thanks to Dr. Ann Lucas who provided photos and also kindly read our manuscript; and to Ken Levinson for his photography.

Thanks also to: Dr. Donald Abt, Associate Dean of the University of Pennsylvania's School of Veterinary Medicine; Michael Walters, Public Information Director of the American Veterinary Medical Association; Dr. Jacqueline Matzler, Ph.D. in Neuroscience and student at the University of Pennsylvania's School of Veterinary Medicine; Elaine Newton, Director of Public Relations, The Society for Prevention of Cruelty to Animals; Deborah Derickson, Public Relations Manager, the Zoological Society of Philadelphia; to Ginny Clemens for her super *Superanimals*; Dorothy Litchfield and her sister, Eleanor Litchfield, for their enthusiasm and professional interest; to Fran Accetta and her daughter Jill for typing and posing for photos.

Finally, to our son Rick and daughters Barbara and Monica our thanks for their continuing encouragement of our career.

Mary Price Lee
Richard S. Lee

CONTENTS

DEDICATION

For Lee, Dorothy, Mary Wynne and Pearl

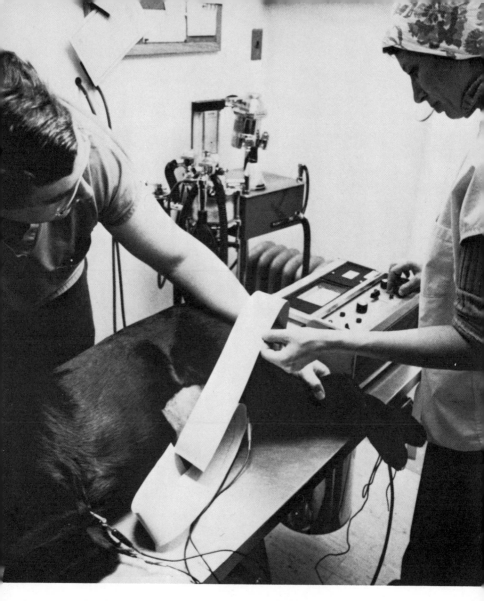

Dr. Lucas (right) may include an electrocardiogram (EKG) in her examination. Photo: Ken Levinson.

CHAPTER 1

ANIMAL CARE CAREERS MARCH WITH THE TIMES

In the 1970s, the traditional animal care career areas—*veterinary medicine, animal welfare work, animal training*—dominated the field. Today that field has expanded to include almost as many career areas as the leopard has spots. *Preventive medicine, computer applications, environmental concerns,* and many other developments have penetrated the animal care field and enlarged its scope.

PREVENTIVE MEDICINE

Dr. Donald Abt, Associate Dean of the University of Pennsylvania School of Veterinary Medicine, says that veterinary medicine has traditionally emphasized preventive care. Doctors in small animal practice and in equine (horse) medicine have encouraged owners to provide their animals with preventive inoculations and nutritionally balanced diets.

While economic factors are not usually related to the purpose of preventive medicine, Dr. Abt explains that there is one area recently in which preventive medicine and finances relate. The main purpose of the recent trend in *cattle herd programs* is to increase productivity and raise health levels through preventive medicine. The herd programs provide many new jobs, for instance, in controlling and eliminating the disease mastitis, keeping detailed records of fertility cycles, calving dates and immunizations to create model herds—and enhance the breeders' return on their investments.

COMPUTERIZATION OF THE FIELD

The computer did not bypass veterinary medicine as it revolutionized the business world. Today, small and large animal practitioners use personal computers to maintain medical records and financial balance sheets. Computer-based diagnostic systems are used in many large animal hospitals; they help veterinary surgeons and assistants in pinpointing medical problems, and often refer them to other sources of information on a given medical subject.

CARE AND CONSERVATION OF WILDLIFE

Veterinarians and other animal health care people have new advocates in the increasing numbers of people in our country who have become newly aware of the need for wildlife care and conservation. Until recently, only small, special-interest groups expressed concern over birds and animals lost to declining natural habitats or disappearing because of ecological damage. Now, hundreds of thousands of caring citizens are aware that healthy wildlife is both a humane goal and a necessity if the balance of nature is to be preserved. With this growing support and publicity, more workers in animal care have recently been able to make *wildlife preservation* and *conservation* their specialties.

PETS AND PSYCHOLOGY

Another current trend is the preoccupation with fitness. These are *holistic* times, dedicated to the well-being of the whole person. Personal fulfillment, contentment and a healthy mind are concerns that share attention with top physical condition. This concern for fitness extends to animal care. Today, there are *pet psychologists*; neurotic animal behavior can be painstakingly treated in frequent visits to a specialized pet doctor.

When pets are not being analyzed themselves, they may be providing comfort as companions to the aged, as anchors to reality for the mentally disturbed, or as an incentive to action for the physically impaired. "Dumb animal" is simply not an accurate appraisal when one witnesses the miracles that can occur between pet and human. *Animal ecologists* (another growing specialty) have discovered that animals have a special sensitivity to the needs and problems of handicapped people, a seemingly obvious idea that only recently has been recognized. The therapeutic value of pets gives an additional meaning to the word *companion* in *companion animal*—the animal care professional's phrase for pets.

THE VETERINARY ASSISTANT

The sharing of professional responsibilities formerly exercised almost entirely by the veterinarian has led to new and satisfying jobs in the animal field. Paralegal and paramedical assistants have been around for many years, but the appearance of the *paraveterinary specialist* is relatively recent (the title is generally *veterinary assistant* or *veterinary technician* rather than paraveterinary, but the functions and duties are equivalent). The veterinary assistant now has far more complex

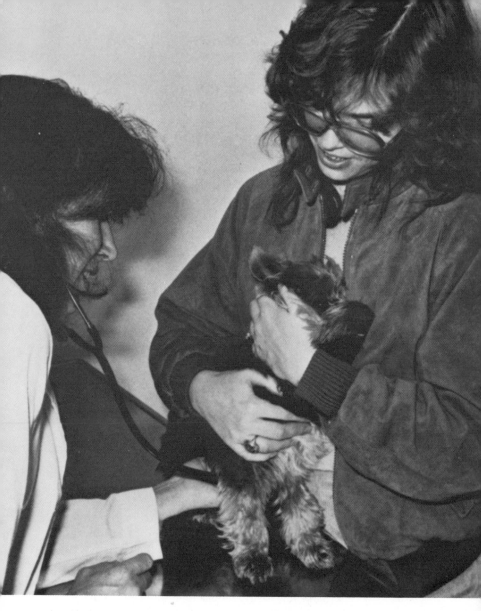

Dr. Lucas starts every visit with a physical exam. Photo: Ken Levinson.

assignments than the usual routine animal care chores. Surgical preparation, emergency first aid, and the basics of preventive medicine are among the many duties performed by these qualified specialists.

The roll-call of fields and specialties within animal care continues to grow each year. From *animal ambulance driver* to *pet bereavement counselor,* total animal care is a priority of this decade, and beyond.

This is good news for you. It means more jobs, greater choice, and more opportunity to enter this worthy field, and create a life-long career. While many positions may be somewhat hard to come by now, the popularity of animal care and an increasing realization of its importance is creating new opportunities.

•

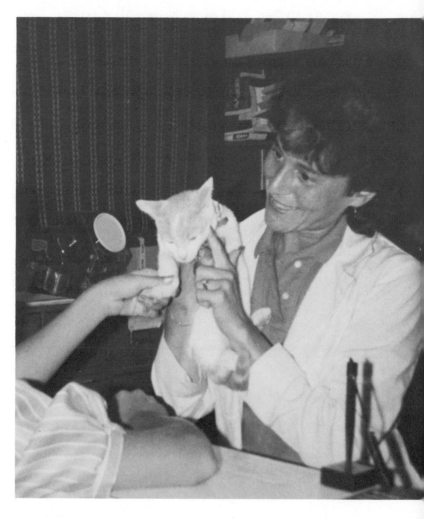

Owner Jill Accetta entrusts her cat to the veterinarian. Photo: M. P. Lee, R. S. Lee.

CHAPTER 2

ANIMAL CARE HISTORY: FROM MAGIC TO MEDICAL EXPERTISE, FROM EXPLOITATION TO PROTECTION

Magic was the earliest form of medical treatment for humans and animals alike. Practitioners called upon the supernatural to cure all their patients! Fortunately, medicine is now based on the scientific method instead of incantations.

VETERINARY MEDICINE IN ANCIENT TIMES

Veterinary medicine is as old as civilization. Early people in the Mediterranean lands began to domesticate animals and to turn from a hunting to an agricultural society at least 4,000 years B.C. A veterinary profession developed throughout large parts of Africa and Asia, to tend animals that sickened. The Egyptians, Babylonians and Hindus all developed human and animal medicine as one practice, while the early Greeks developed the scientific method and taught animal and human anatomy.

The Babylonians are credited with a significant early step in animal medicine, the isolation of sick animals from the herd.

Although ailing animals were treated by magic, these early animal doctors passed the isolation technique on to the Hebrews who in turn passed on the idea to later Western civilizations.

By the beginning of the second century B.C., veterinary practice had taken root in the agrarian society of India where cattle were the most valuable resource. The Hindu religious concept of reincarnation—and with it the sacred status of the cow—was the basis for serious concern about animal care. India continued to develop animal care, establishing veterinary hospitals in the Middle Ages. Even today, there are government-operated *gosadans* (literally "old cow homes") that are a direct outgrowth of these early veterinary hospitals.

The Greeks were the first people to record detailed veterinary history. In 400 B.C., King Alexander of Macedonia created programs of animal study, and the Greek physician, Hippocrates, recognized the similarities between animal and human physiology as he plunged into the exciting sciences of pathology and anatomy. Over 200 years later, Galen, a Greek physician working in Rome, dissected horses and noted his anatomical and physiological observations. *The Hippiatrika,* the first detailed veterinary writing, was developed in the Byzantine Empire by Aspyrtus and Vegetius, acknowledged as the true founders of veterinary medicine.

A TIME OF DARKNESS

From the fall of the Roman Empire until the Renaissance, much medical information, human and animal, was lost. However, the horseshoe was invented during this time, and the *farrier* (or shoer of horses) was the nearest thing to a veterinarian. The horse was one of the few animals in this period that was medically studied. In fact, in 1598, a veterinary work, *The*

Anatomy of the Horse, was published. It was a detailed study, although crude by today's standards.

Another scholar, the Benedictine Abbess, St. Hildegarde, was also at work during this period, and prepared a study on animals, fish, and birds. She did not draw from earlier studies of any sort, but gathered voluminous information herself.

The Renaissance arrived to waken an intellectually slumbering world, and among its contributions was a revival of interest in medicine. Advances in the control of human and animal diseases were due in large part to the discovery of the circulation of the blood and the invention of the microscope.

At this time, people were studying animals in different ways. In the late 15th Century, an early zoo was created on the grounds of the Regent of France, Anne de Beaujeu. This curious monarch raised animals in the stately gardens behind the Royal Palace. She also studied the habits of turkeys, an unseemly pastime for aristocrats of the period!

ANIMAL CARE IN FRANCE

It was not until 1762 that animal care in Europe was organized into a formal tradition. This development was prompted by a devastating cattle plague that begged for a hasty solution. As a result, the first veterinary college, Ecole Nationale Vétérinaire of Lyons, France, was formed. The college attempted to find ways to combat the plague by methods other than quarantine and slaughter.

Less than one hundred years later, the French physician and scientist, Louis Pasteur, discovered micro-organisms, and established their relationship to diseases in people and other animals. Pasteur's studies encouraged veterinarians to protect animals from communicable diseases. The doctor's interest extended also to protecting humans from diseases of animal origin, particularly those transmitted through meats and dairy products. The principles of food hygiene begun in the 19th Century owe much to Pasteur's trailblazing research.

RURAL AMERICA

The first stirrings of animal health care in America revolved around a directive, *Liberties of Brute Animals*. The Puritans of the Massachusetts Bay Colony wrote the treatise, a voluntary set of rules governing humane animal care.

It was still to be more than 200 years before any general animal welfare movement would surface in America; yet between 1650 and 1850 there developed the rudiments of veterinary medicine, and a gradual separation of the field from human medicine.

People shipping animals to America—early America counted heavily on cattle, swine and horses from abroad—had their own way of keeping a disease from spreading. The crews of the animal-laden ships were directed to toss any sick animals overboard. Although a heartless process, this practice prevented at least some of the livestock contamination caused by imported stock.

In these formative years of a developing country, wildlife was considered every citizen's property, to be consumed without restriction or governmental control. Commercial demand for leather, fur, feathers, and meat led to wholesale exploitation of wild animals. Domestic cattle succumbed to disease rather than greed as anthrax, pleuropneumonia, and hog cholera were increasingly prevalent.

Two events within a year of each other meant hope for both wildlife and livestock. *The Morrill Land Grant Act of 1862* was passed by Congress, providing federal land and funds for education in agriculture, the mechanical arts, and veterinary science. A year later, the *American Veterinary Medical Association* was founded. Its aim was a full-scale attack on the diseases of domestic livestock. Only in more recent years has this organization been able to concentrate on total care for all animals. In 1884, Congress passed the *Hatch Act,* landmark legislation that established the *Bureau of Animal Industry* within the *U.S. Department of Agriculture.* The Bureau regulated the importation of cattle in order to control contagious pleuropneumonia, the most persistent cattle disease, and other livestock illnesses.

EARLY HUMANE AND CONSERVATION EFFORTS

While there was some enlightenment in the field, cruelty to animals and indifference to their plight were still "givens." Many horses were treated as cruelly in fact as "Black Beauty" was in fiction. At one time in New York City alone, some 25,000 horses, many drawing streetcars, were poorly cared for and overworked. Henry Bergh, a wealthy New York career diplomat, left the diplomatic service to devote his life to curtailing animal cruelty among the hapless horses and other creatures. In a ringing speech delivered on February 8, 1886, Bergh declared that "...the blood-red hand of cruelty shall no longer torture dumb animals with impunity." On that day, Bergh established the *American Society for the Prevention of Cruelty to Animals (ASPCA).*

Bergh also pressed for the enactment of the *Animal Welfare Act of 1886* in New York State. Under its terms, any act of animal cruelty was a misdemeanor with specific penalties. It shortly became the model for legislation in other states. Only six days after the Act was passed, a Brooklyn butcher piled sheep and calves into a cart like so many bags of grain. The butcher was the first of a parade of violators that year to feel the sting of the new animal protection law.

The following year, a national federation of animal welfare agencies was established in an effort to make welfare programs more unified among the growing number of independent agencies. The move was the beginning of a concerted effort to treat *all* animals like people's best friends.

While humane societies arose to do their part, health education in the animal field was also expanding. More than 22 colleges were offering courses in veterinary subjects. The first public veterinary college was begun at Iowa State College. Today, there are 27 colleges of veterinary medicine in the United States and three in Canada. Of the early private institutions of veterinary medicine, only the University of Pennsylvania remains.

For twenty years before 1883, Americans were gradually becoming more aware of the finite nature of wildlife. Spurred by the writings of James Audubon, John Muir, Henry Thoreau and John Burroughs, people were forming conservation organizations. Since these early efforts posed no threat to industry, they were tolerated. (To a degree, this perspective continues today.) But by 1883, fewer than 1,000 of America's onetime bison population of 60 million remained; fur-bearing animals were in danger of extinction; the passenger pigeon was nearly gone—it would disappear forever in 1914. *The American Ornithologists Union,* founded in 1883, was the first national conservation group; others like the *Sierra Club* (1892) and the *New York Zoological Society* were founded. This latter organization was the first dedicated to wildlife conservation as we understand it today.

TODAY

There is a growing interrelationship among the many groups concerned with animal preservation and animal care. The connection between humans and animals long separated in veterinary medicine has merged as well. Veterinary medicine has taken an increasingly active role in researching the medical uses of atomic energy, in the application of many drugs with common uses for people and animals, in the research efforts of the space program, and in the control and elimination of zoonoses (ailments common to humans and animals). Veterinarians now interact with agricultural specialists as well, in their common concern for food purity as it relates to animal drugs and animal feed pesticides.

In this capsule history, we have not traced the important contributions to animal care made by *zoological societies*. Zoos have evolved from places of animal confinement to habitats designed for the understanding and the protection of endangered species, and for the education of people in the importance of preserving the balance of nature. Author-zoologists such as Lawrence Durrell actively promote this essential element of animal care through numerous highly readable books, and through the protectionist work performed by his Isle of Jersey Zoo off the English coast.

The tremendous growth of the American pet population provides this final historical note: there are more than 2,000 animal welfare organizations in the country today, ranging from small local SPCA's to national groups. The tremendous pet population has also ushered in a broad range of pet care services, from dog grooming salons to operating amphitheaters for animal shows. Many new animal care occupations offer career opportunities today that did not exist even a few years ago.

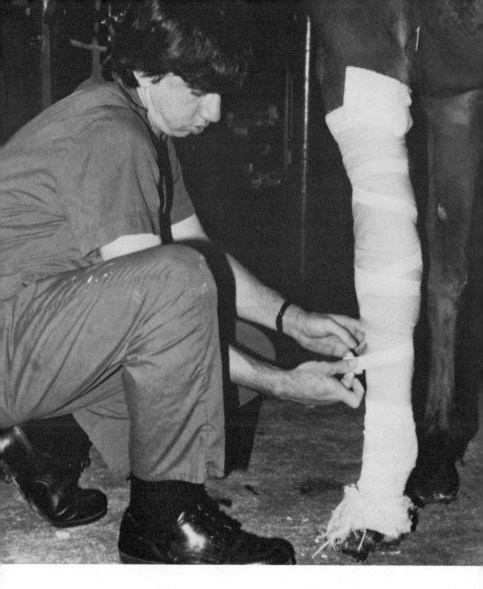

An injured leg can be treated in many cases today, though it once meant death for large animals like horses. Photo: University of Illinois College of Veterinary Medicine.

THE TURN OF THE CENTURY—
INCREASING CONCERN FOR ANIMALS

The first half of the 20th Century saw the establishment of state and federal wildlife agencies designed to promote the careful use of natural resources including wildlife. During this time, eradication of diseases continued to be the primary goal of veterinary medicine. Toward mid-century, especially after World War II, veterinarians began a greater degree of interaction with human medical specialists and increased their involvement with control and protection of the pet population—characteristics of today's veterinary practice and animal medical research.

In the early years of the 1930's, Alfred Leopold, a professional forester, began to formulate ecological and evolutionary theories. He recognized the existence of "ecosystems," the interdependence of human beings, animals and environment. By mid-decade, Leopold was questioning the validity of prevailing wildlife management concepts that favored certain species. While game animals received the major share of attention, predatory animals remained "second-class citizens."

A major spur to the conservation movement was Rachel Carson's book, *Silent Spring*. In it, the author demonstrated the dangers of current practices such as insecticide use and destruction of wildlife and its habitat for commercial purposes. The conservation awareness she generated led to the formation of the *Environmental Protection Agency, the President's Council on Environmental Quality* and promoted the enactment of the *Wilderness Act, Endangered Species Act* and *National Environmental Policy Act*. A not-so-gentle ripple had grown to a strong current of concern—and this time, a woman was proving the pen to be mightier than the sword.

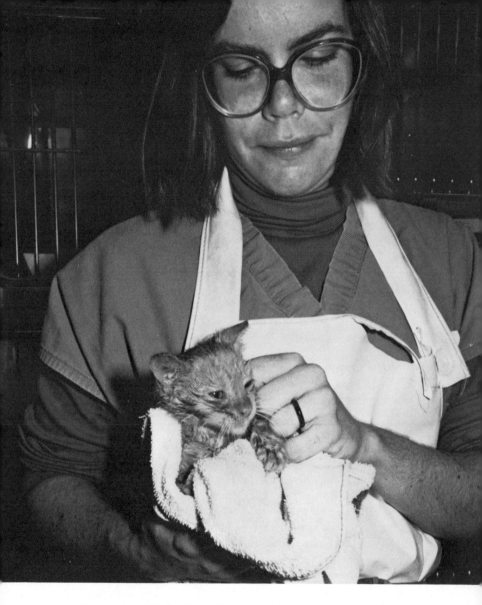

Grooming includes bathing, nail clipping, hair trimming and conditioning.
Photo: Ken Levinson.

CHAPTER 3

HAVING THAT "SPECIAL SOMETHING" FOR WORK IN ANIMAL CARE: PATIENCE, WARMTH AND RESPECT FOR LIVING CREATURES

We as a nation have an ongoing love affair with animals. Americans own and care for 48 million dogs, 25 million cats, 23 million birds, 12 million exotic pets—and 340 million fish!

Although many of us enjoy and appreciate animals, making them your career calls for a "special something." It includes two vital elements: *aptitude* and *attitude*.

APTITUDE FOR ANIMAL CARE CAREERS

Among the elements of aptitude you will need are robust good health—animal care is physically and mentally demanding, far from the glamorous work too often portrayed in the media. Ministering to an ailing horse may be an around-the-clock job. Placing radio transmitters on hibernating black bears to track their later movements will call for wilderness survival skills as well as physical strength and a high degree of courage.

Whether you are rescuing ducks from an oil spill, changing cat cages in a veterinary clinic or training dogs for the show ring, your aptitude must include an almost inborn affinity for animals, an ability to handle them where others could not approach, a knowledge of their habits coupled with a lack of fear of the animals in your care, a calm competence that they can sense about you. With these attributes comes an almost instinctive appreciation of an animal's weaknesses coupled with a healthy respect for its strengths and its unpredictability.

You may already know how well you get along with animals; but if your aspirations outweigh your experience in this important respect, you should make every effort to see if your love of animals translates into an ability to manage them. This self-testing must go beyond owning and caring for a pet or two. A summer's work in some area of animal care should tell you whether it is the field for you.

ATTITUDE—EQUALLY ESSENTIAL

With few exceptions, high income does not exist in animal care any more than glamour does. These are among the most giving of careers, in which the desire to be of help to your fellow-creatures (we are all animals!) outweighs considerations of comfort, physical, or material.

This altruism—of doing good as you see it in an animal context—is a key element in the attitude you need for fulfillment of your career. But it is not the only element. Your emotional attachment to animals must be tempered with professionalism if you are to maintain a healthy balance in your work. The anger you may face at seeing an injury or injustice done to an animal must be tempered with the knowledge of what to do, and with the degree of professional objectivity needed to do it.

Without this coolness under fire, you cannot function in a helpful way.

Your attitude must be the result of having come to grips with moral and ethical judgments as well as emotions. Although animals have rights, as the Humane Society of the United States has made clear, they are nevertheless viewed as "products" in a society that depends on many of them for food. They are also viewed as necessary elements of biological and human medical research. New drugs and medical devices cannot be approved for human use until their effectiveness has been proven on animal subjects. Animal shelter employees must constantly deal with the hard facts of euthanasia—"good death" is the Greek meaning for the humane disposition of ill or unwanted animals. Veterinarians and their helpers must cope daily with animal illness and death. These are facts of life; they cannot be changed. Your moral convictions cannot be at war with your work if you are to be happy in it. If you can see the necessity of animals as food products, you may find great personal satisfaction in research designed to improve the health of livestock, or in seeing that such animals are raised and handled under humane conditions. This applies equally well to supervising laboratory animals—if you feel that their uses in the testing of medical innovations is a necessary part of improving the quality of life for society.

Your attitude, therefore, must agree with the one prevailing in your workplace. Let's say you are the conservation-minded Assistant Curator of Mammals at a zoo. If the zoo is one where animal health is enhanced and endangered species are nurtured, you will be happy in the contribution you make to these goals. If on the other hand the zoo for which you work exists primarily for the amusement of visitors rather than for a higher purpose, you would soon become disenchanted with its policies.

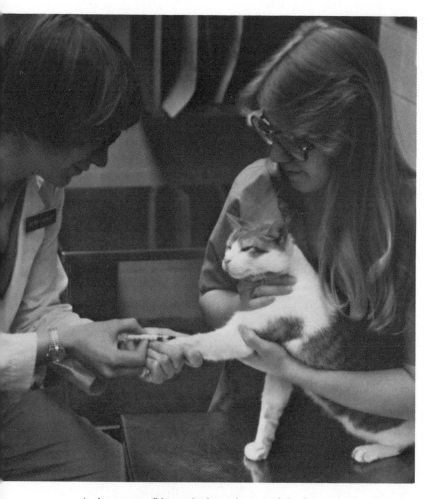

A pleasant, confident attitude on the part of the doctor reassures the nervous pet owner. Photo: Michigan State University, College of Veterinary Medicine, Animal Technology Program and North American Veterinary Technicians Association.

INTERLOCKING OF APTITUDE AND ATTITUDE

It's almost self-evident, then, that aptitude and attitude will interrelate in the well-adjusted animal care careerist. Together, they constitute your basic approach to your career.

Much of your aptitude—the ability to relate to animals, your physical stamina, ability to learn, and acceptance of less than great financial rewards—will be reinforced by your attitude: positive, cheerful, calm in the face of frustration, professional in your acceptance of reality. With such an approach, your rewards will be self-esteem and continued pleasure in a lifetime spent with animals.

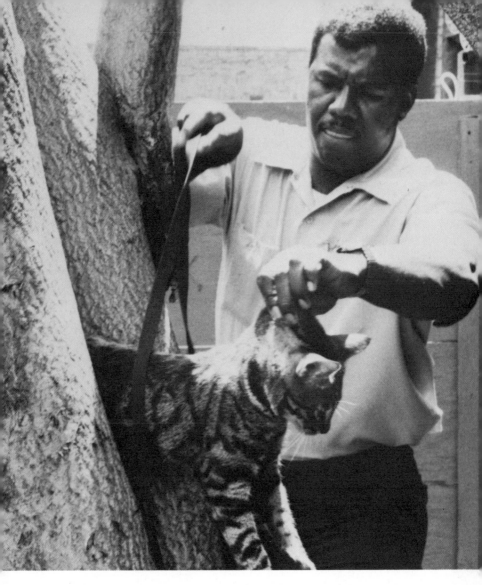

A Pennsylvania SPCA (Society for the Prevention of Cruelty to Animals) shelter supervisor extracts a cat from the fork of a tree. Photo: Pennsylvania SPCA.

CHAPTER 4

VOLUNTEERING AND APPRENTICESHIP—AN ANSWER TO JOB MARKET UNCERTAINTIES

Currently almost two million people are directly or indirectly involved with animals. These employment figures would seem to show animal care as a healthy field. Alas, not all the news is good.

THE ANIMAL CARE EMPLOYMENT OUTLOOK

Everything favors general job opportunity in the animal care field. Never before has there been such an interest in animal conservation and enlightened animal care. Paralleling this movement is a trend to return to the land and its creatures. This urban retreat should spell jobs for individuals in animal medicine, in humane care work, in wildlife and range specialties and in areas of self-employment. (The enthusiastic horse-woman, for instance, may make her living raising thorough-breds, racing them, stabling horses for others and giving riding lessons.)

Although positions in the U.S. Fish & Wildlife Service have doubled and jobs at the Humane Society of the United States have increased fourfold, positions in some animal care areas are hard to come by. The reason is there are simply more people attracted to the field than there are jobs for them. This interest often begins in childhood and for many continues into adulthood; unfortunately, in some career areas where jobs may not be plentiful.

Some of the chapters on individual animal careers will detail the job market for that particular field, but a few generalizations are possible here. They will illustrate the differences between job expectations and job availabilities. For instance, there are many laboratory animal clinician positions available as veterinary assistant, humane society health technician, or working in the more rarefied atmosphere of animal research. A profession such as zoology is less promising, but is holding its own. This field encompasses such a broad area that while some specialties may be overcrowded, others offer job opportunities. Among their many duties, zoologists study animals in their natural habitats the world over, collect specimens for laboratory study, and study animal diseases.

One of the less promising employment areas is animal conservation including range management. Despite strong national interest and the creation of a greater number of jobs, vast legions of workers striving to protect wildlife and save endangered species is just a mirage. (The U.S. Government's Occupational Handbook for 1982 does state, however, that demand for range managers may increase as legislators vote funds to carry out the wishes of the very strong conservation lobby.) These jobs are generally within federal and state jurisdictions. Openings only occur when someone moves *on* or *out*.

WAYS TO GET A JOB
IN A HIGHLY COMPETITIVE FIELD

There are many ways to pursue and *secure* a job in these popular fields of animal care—even the ones difficult to enter. Make sure first of all that you have the specialized education needed for your field. Then build on this academic cornerstone with practical experience. Volunteer work, an apprenticeship and workshops all offer hands-on education.

Guy Hodge, Director, Research and Data, of the Humane Society of the United States, feels that on-the-job training gives the prospective animal care worker the edge. You get to know the management—those people who may be able to give you a helping hand later. You may also learn about job openings before they "go public," and be able to declare yourself eligible.

THE MANY WAYS TO VOLUNTEER

The on-the-job training that Guy Hodge so strongly recommends is best achieved by volunteer work. Volunteering comes in many forms: assisting in a pet shop; volunteering for national park work; or just working on your own in some helpful way with animals.

VOLUNTEERING IN SPCAs,
VETERINARY OFFICES, AND ZOOS

High schoolers and college students with summers free are often welcome to pitch in at busy SPCAs, community zoos or veterinary offices. Generally, volunteer work in such places involves the rock-bottom chores like cleaning cages and feeding endless corridors of noisy, demanding creatures. But such chores are performed by almost *everyone* in the animal care field at one time or another. Even managers of local zoos may find themselves doing shovel-duty on a day when a keeper calls in sick. It's good training, then, to learn from the ground up— literally—how to keep animal surroundings clean!

VOLUNTEERING OPPORTUNITIES IN THE WILDLIFE FIELD

Another volunteer avenue may lead to your local nature center. (City residents may be surprised that nature centers often fall within the city limits, or not far beyond them.) If there is a local chapter of the Audubon Society or its equivalent, find out from them what you can do to help. Another similar area devoted to wildlife study and preservation would be your city's natural sciences academy. (A good part of Boston's Science Museum, for instance, is devoted to wild animal study and display. Philadelphia has a separate—and very large— Academy of Natural Sciences.)

If these places have no room for you as a volunteer, they can still be helpful. Classes, weekend outings and "sightings" will make you more knowledgeable and thus more comfortable with your subject. Membership in a nature center, natural sciences museum or zoo will reduce the costs and make you a part of these special, animal-related activities.

The volunteer programs of the National Park Service currently have 9,000 people at work in Park Service facilities. Volunteers may help give tours, lectures, or lend a hand managing a site. Young people under age 18 must have parental permission and may find out other particulars from their National Park Service Regional Office.

The National Forest Program has 15,000 industrious volunteers, too, and information on volunteer work may be obtained from any national forest headquarters. There is no payment for work, but the tab for uniforms, lodging and transportation is generally picked up by the U.S. Government, the parent organization.

The Student Conservation Association places high school and college students in National Park and National Forest areas, where they may meet the problems of conservation head-on. Guy Hodge's book, "Careers: Working With Animals—the Humane Society's Guide" notes that those interested may write The Student Conservation Association, Box 440, Charlestown, NH 03603.

If you live in the country near woods or grasslands, you can devote time to learning about wildlife on your own. While you cannot set up a wildlife shelter, develop educational programs or provide incubators for baby owls (you usually need a state permit to do these things), you can study owls, racoons, squirrels, birds and other wildlife in their natural environments and report cases of cruelty or abandonment to humane societies.

You may even have to report do-gooders—well-meaning families who try to tame wild creatures. They often do great harm, causing stress in an unnatural environment and depriving the animal of its natural nutrition.

Ms. Mary Ann Williams of Newtown, Pennsylvania, is a wildlife *advocate,* a person whose goal is to return injured or abandoned wildlife to the wilderness. While some of her time is taken educating the public through school and community lectures, most of her effort goes into helping wild creatures back on their feet, or up and away on their wings. Her volunteer center aided more than 600 animals in a recent year, from foxes to Canada Geese—such activity definitely out-McDonalds Old

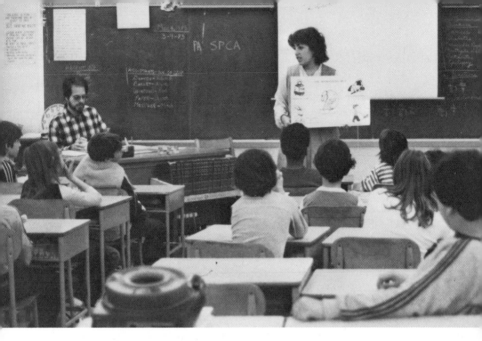

SPCA volunteers distribute literature about animal and pet care in the schools and at many public gatherings. Photo: Pennsylvania SPCA.

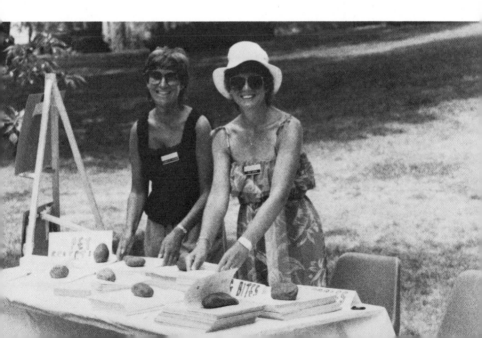

McDonald's Farm! Her work is highly respected, and although it is not reinforced with a paycheck, she has surely found herself *the* job of a lifetime.

THE 4-H CLUBS AND FUTURE FARMERS

The four Hs of the 4-H Clubs stand for Head, Heart, Hands and Health. Actually, there should be another H, for Helping. Helping for free—or volunteering—is what 4-H Clubs are all about. Children bake the cookies to sell to help an ailing neighbor; adults volunteer to do the carpentry for the 4-H carnival booths.

Ask a sampling of people what 4-H Clubs are all about, and they'll probably say "agriculture." They are right, in part. Farming and animal-raising play strong roles in 4-H activities, just as they do in Future Farmers of America chapters. While FFA concentrates on farm crops and farm animals, today's 4-H Club members may also be learning about textiles, hair styling or computers.

Still, the rural image persists in both organizations, along with their involvement with animals. For instance, some 4-H chapters sponsor Seeing Eye Puppy Clubs. Pups are given to 4-H youngsters to raise for a year. These dogs go everywhere with their families—to the store, on trips and other places where their future blind owners may go. When the year is up, the dog is ready for formal training and placement as a lead dog. (Ask the 4-H Club near you if they have such a program, or others that involve working with animals. There are 4-H Clubs throughout the country.)

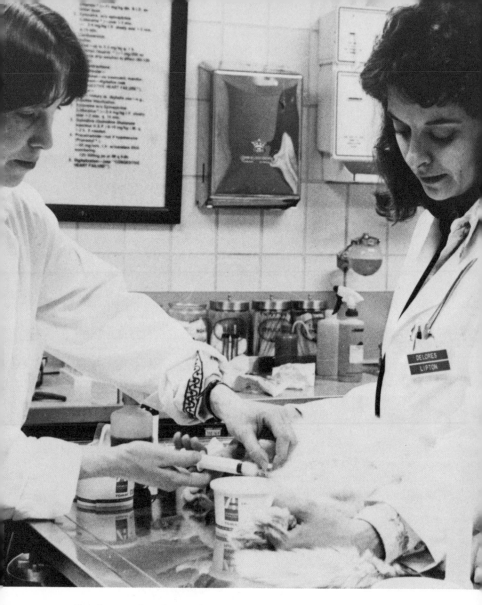

Veterinary students have to learn to give injections. Photo: University of Illinois College of Veterinary Medicine.

CHAPTER 5

FROM INTERESTED TEEN TO FULL-FLEDGED VET: THE ROUTE TO A DVM DEGREE

If you want to be a veterinarian, now is the time to start planning. *Now* is if you're 13, 16, or even in college. This chapter will give you the academic low-down—the courses you'll want to take to be in line for a place in veterinary medicine.

JUNIOR HIGH AND HIGH SCHOOL

Junior High is the time when sciences seem to overtake other subjects on your roster. This is just fine. Take what is offered and you'll find this knowledge becomes the cornerstone of your senior high school science curriculum. High school science courses—biology, mathematics, chemistry and physics—are *musts*. Although you may think they are heavy going, they are merely a lighthearted introduction to the rigorous science program college pre-vets must face.

Although this chapter is mainly about the necessary academics, there are some other important preparatory steps for a veterinary career. Caring for neighbors' pets, attending local and state animal fairs and school science fairs, joining the local 4-H Club or Future Farmers (see Chapter 4 for more on this) and visiting a veterinary school open house if you live near one of the schools of veterinary medicine, will all help you in your chosen career. In addition to giving you a taste of your future work, activities such as these will be looked-on favorably by the colleges to which you apply.

CHOOSING A COLLEGE

You should take ample time to choose a college that will prepare you for veterinary school. It may be helpful to consider the possibility of attending a college with a veterinary school. You will have access to the veterinary school faculty (they sometimes teach undergraduate science courses) and to animal care clubs. The science courses you take as an undergraduate will very likely reflect the philosophy of the veterinary school. But if you cannot attend a college or university with a veterinary school, your chances of entering veterinary school will be diminished little if at all. Your grades, your college's academic standards, and that important consideration, your personality and affinity for the field, will ultimately decide the issue.

Colleges offer you a great opportunity to turn aspirations into accomplishments. In short, study hard. Top grades *do* count because of the tremendous pressure to get into veterinary school. Extracurricular activities begun in your high school years should be continued and expanded; pre-veterinary club work, SPCA work (paid or volunteer), summer work on a farm or in a veterinary hospital will help increase your chances of admission to veterinary school.

COLLEGE CURRICULUM

Besides a well-rounded program in communications skills and social sciences, pre-veterinary students should spend a large segment of undergraduate time in the sciences. Zoology, botany, physical chemistry and physiology coupled with extensive lab periods will provide a concentrated undergraduate experience in the sciences.

Pre-veterinary students generally complete their undergraduate studies and receive their Bachelor of Science Degrees before entering veterinary school for another four-year program. But there are variations on this pattern that you might want to consider. Some colleges connected with veterinary schools offer a Bachelor of Science Degree in Pre-Veterinary Medicine that is awarded after three years of undergraduate work and completion of the first year of veterinary school. For some students this degree may be sufficient for animal care careers that do not need the credentials of the full-fledged DVM.

CHOOSING A VETERINARY SCHOOL

Although the number of schools offering veterinary medicine has increased to a more equitable 27 (with three in Canada), competition for a Freshman spot is still fierce. The acceptance rate is about 42% of the total number applying. In fact, it is more difficult to qualify for veterinary school than for medical school because there are far fewer of them. The popularity of veterinary medicine has helped swell the number of applicants.

Geographical limitations can pose problems that you should investigate. Many states have no veterinary schools. Under a contract system, veterinary school applicants in these states apply to schools in neighboring states. Seldom is a resident of a state accepted by a veterinary school that has no admissions contract with that state. Because veterinary schools must accept qualified students from their own states and honor contracts with adjoining states, the whole acceptance procedure can be as complex as a chess game. However, there has been a definite easing of restrictions in this area; entrance is not as difficult as it has been. Nevertheless, the problems should be addressed as they may apply to the state in which you live, and the veterinary school you wish to enter.

COST OF VETERINARY SCHOOL

Once enrolled you are not home free—literally! The cost of a veterinary medical education today can be astounding. While some veterinary colleges can keep costs down because of state subsidies, other colleges will cost from $45,000 to $60,000 for your four years of tuition, room and board. And a rule of thumb: it is very expensive for a student to go out-of-state for his or her veterinary education. Veterinary students in financial need can borrow up to $3,500 a year from the federal government under the provisions of the Veterinary Medical Education Act and Health Manpower Act of 1968.

A more realistic cost appraisal is about $3,000 a year for a state-supported school and $7,000 and up for private colleges, room and board excluded. Scholarships, loans and grants can reduce these burdens, of course.

It doesn't take a math whiz to see that the return on your investment will be a long time in coming. If you as a DVM with $40,000 in education debts take a job paying $22,000, you will be a few years in putting yourself in the black. If you're entering private practice, your school debt could be at least doubled by your start-up needs. This topic is covered more in Chapter 7.

It would help, of course, if you could meet undergraduate payments and start your career free of debt. But as Dr. Donald Abt mentions, you do not go into veterinary medicine for the money. It is a profession that attracts a specific kind of person for a most unusual field. That is not to say that ultimately it cannot prove financially rewarding.

Dr. Robert Marshak, Dean of the School of Veterinary Medicine of the University of Pennsylvania, defends the high costs. Medical school clinics, he explains, enjoy revenues from patients and reimbursement from health insurers. Veterinary medicine has no such remuneration. Dr. Marshak further explains that veterinary medicine is more complex and thus more costly. This is because it deals with different species. Human medicine does not confront animals who differ in the number of stomachs they may have (the cow, for instance, has four stomach-like compartments). Such variations require different kinds of equipment, a greater diagnostic ability, even different kinds of hospitals.

YOUR VETERINARY SCHOOL EXPERIENCE

Assuming you're accepted and confident that you can make it financially, what is in store for you in your four years? For most veterinary students, graduate school is an exhausting, exhilarating time that can only be eclipsed by work in the actual field itself.

The first two years are mostly spent in-house as the veterinary student comes to grips with the basic medical sciences. Anatomy, biochemistry, microbiology, physiology and pharmacology are among the scientific mainstays. Students learn the normal characteristics of the many types of animals as applied to these disciplines and then study the changes that come from disease and injury. This introductory period could aptly be

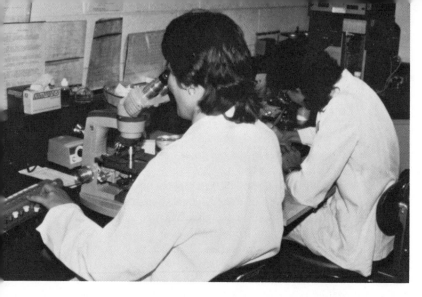

Veterinary training involves both clinical and research experience. Photos: upper, Michigan State University, College of Veterinary Medicine, Animal Technology Program and North American Veterinary Technician Association; lower, University of Illinois College of Veterinary Medicine.

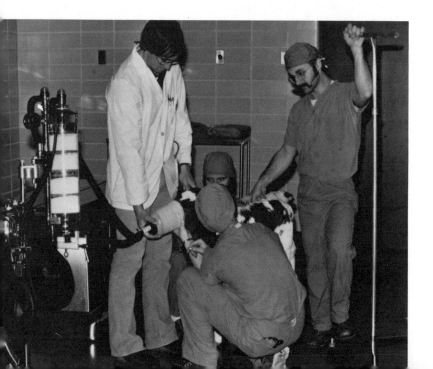

called "Noah's Ark in Sickness and in Health." (For summer experience, get in touch with the U.S. Department of Agriculture. They regularly hire veterinary students during the summer months.)

The final two years offer hands-on experience. Animal clinic work, laboratory periods and classes in life-work areas such as veterinary law and public health services prepare the veterinary student for the real world of animal medicine.

The typical day of a fourth-year student may go like this: clinic work starts the round of activities, beginning as early as 7:30 A.M. Life can be frantic in this post-dawn period. Cases are admitted, histories are taken and blood work is prepared. By early afternoon, things may quiet down, but surgery often highlights the afternoon agenda. Evenings may be free (for study, of course), but then again, the student who started at 7:30 A.M. may have night duty as well.

Not all days are equally hectic. Classwork and library research are the other end of the spectrum. Both the excitement and the scholarly calm add up to a veterinarian in the making. It's a matter of time—four years, in fact—before the hard-working veterinary student becomes a qualified (and equally hard-working) Doctor of Veterinary Medicine.

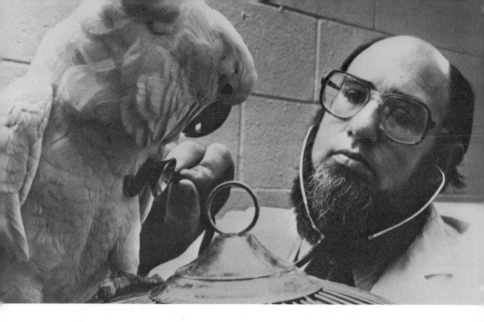

Veterinarians can choose what type of animals they want to work with—
large or small. Photo: upper, Zoological Society of Pennsylvania; lower,
Michigan State University, College of Veterinary Medicine, Animal
Technology Program and North American Veterinary Technicians
Association.

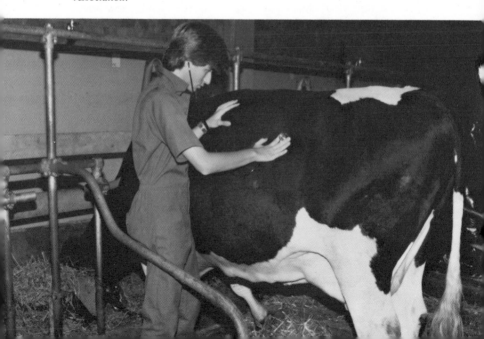

CHAPTER 6

VETERINARY OPTIONS

While medical science can boast of such discoveries as the implanted artificial heart, Veterinary Science has its victories, too. Some are in the medical field, others have social and humanitarian implications. Veterinarians, for instance, are busy finding ways to expand the production of sea creatures so there will be more food for the world's growing population. They are also working to control animal diseases that endanger the world's food supply.

Your interest in veterinary medicine may not extend to social issues; you may wish simply to devote your working life to small animals, or join a zoo staff as resident veterinarian. But "issue person" or not, you will be entering a highly rewarding field.

Veterinary specialties include nearly as many work areas as all other pet care fields combined. With your DVM Degree, you can:

- Run a small animal hospital
- Work in a large animal practice
- Enter public service
- Do research
- Join the military
- Work with zoos

SMALL ANIMAL MEDICINE

If a specialty poll were taken of aspiring veterinarians, most students would want to run or work a small animal hospital. Your decision—to establish your own hospital, join a practice or form a partnership—will depend primarily on your financial situation. (Chapter 7 offers some figures in this area for you to work with.)

Small animal medicine usually involves dogs, cats and other "companion" animals. The animal center for these pets is as important to the immediate neighborhood as the library or the firehouse, and the astute veterinarian-manager-owner gives VIP care. Pets are often registered in such a hospital under their own name (as "Albert" rather than "Mrs. Clark's Dachshund"). Thoughtful touches such as formica examining table tops instead of metal ones (to do away with chill on a pet's feet) are part of the well-run local hospital or clinic.

Private practices today have a new zest as they adopt many of the sophisticated methods of human medicine. Intensive care units are now an established part of many veterinary hospitals. In them, teams rather than single practitioners may work to cure sick animals. One team member of great importance is the veterinary technician. Part nurse, part lab technician, he or she monitors the animal's progress while offering comfort and skilled care. (See Chapter 8.)

Small animal hospitals can vary from the modest office with or without an ICU to the giant, university-connected animal care center. Here, the veterinarian works in three basic areas. He or she *treats, operates* and *advises.* This variety may make life a circus for the veterinarian—or at least a cat-and-dog show.

Variety is evident, too, in the increasing number of specializations veterinarians may enter. In the last fifteen years over twenty specialty fields, neurology and cardiology among them,

have been added to the animal medicine roster. Such sophisticated treatment as open heart surgery, the implanting of electronic pacemakers and chemotherapy are all now a part of
animal medical care. There are also dental veterinarians and
doctors trained to treat the skin diseases of cats and dogs.

A TYPICAL DAY FOR THE VET

For several hours a day, the veterinarian may administer
shots, treat accident victims or give physical examinations.
During other hours (or at any hour if a real emergency arises),
he or she will be in surgery, performing a wide range of operations on sick and injured animals. Because the animals and
their diseases vary, the veterinarian's days are bound to be
different, too.

Consultations are important; the precepts of preventive
medicine are a major part of client appointments. Veterinarians
tell puppy and kitten owners the best routes to health—a good
diet, proper grooming and correct exercise.

Dr. Robin Truelove, a Bethany, Connecticut veterinarian,
starts her work day by visiting her post-op patients or the pets
she has under observation. A puppy may need patching-up after
mixing with a muskrat; a diabetic cat might be next. Before the
morning is over, this busy lady vet may have added a cockatoo
and a poodle to her roll call of patients.

LARGE ANIMAL MEDICINE

Dr. Truelove, a rural resident, is also a large animal practitioner. (Country veterinarians often combine large and small
animal practices.) After fulfilling her morning tasks, she may

head for a local farm, to treat a cow with a stubborn case of mastitis, then check out a horse's infected hoof.

Large animal medicine is also concerned with herd and flock care. Veterinarians may oversee livestock, calving (helping cows give birth), vaccinating herds and charting herd progress. The veterinarian who opts for large animal practice often takes on a whole stable of responsibilities. As he or she travels from farm to farm, this animal doctor must analyze the condition of the farm: its cleanliness and modernity; the personality of its owners (often formidable); the potential of its herds. Large animal practitioners—and these include U.S. Department of Agriculture veterinarians who serve as inspectors—need energy and expertise almost as massive as the herds they oversee.

Pigs, sheep and poultry often qualify as "patients" for large animal practitioners simply because they are farm animals and because their diseases and infirmities can mean financial loss to the farmer and potential danger to neighboring herds. To the caring practitioner, they are as important as the more personable companion animals. For one thing, they have personalities of their own; for another, their medical challenges are important in terms of the veterinarian's professionalism, and of the owner's livelihood.

Large animal practice includes equine care. In fact, the horse plays an important role to many a large animal practitioner. Equine medicine is growing in importance as these valuable animals, including thoroughbred racehorses, receive treatment unavailable just a few years ago. Horse racing, breeding and performance require expert knowledge, and the skilled equine veterinarian can offer advice in both medical and behavioral areas. Whether bred for profit, pleasure or both, the horse has become a focal point of the good life, and its tender loving care is a career for many animal doctors.

A variety of specialties can be found within equine medicine. Besides the thoroughbred and the pleasure pony, there is the role of health inspector for a mounted police unit or for horses going at auction. There is the racetrack veterinarian, too. Equine veterinarians are often surgeons, and some have entered a relatively new sub-specialty, equine sports medicine. The health and performance of the racehorse is the specialty of Dr. William Moyer, Chief Equine Veterinarian at the University of Pennsylvania School of Veterinary Medicine. Dr. Moyer often deals with injuries resulting from the tremendous bursts of speed demanded of racehorses. He works to overcome trauma with techniques such as rehabilitative exercises and whirlpool baths. (Injuries can often be avoided by maintaining good muscle tone and applying therapeutic bandaging.)

Often, racehorses are owned by syndicates; instead of one owner worrying about his half-million-dollar investment, a whole consortium gets ulcers when the horse develops problems. Equine specialists like Dr. Moyer feel this tension, too. In many cases, his worry is not so much the horse as its "family."

PUBLIC SERVICE

The U.S. Department of Agriculture and the Public Health Service (both prime employers of veterinarians) are dedicated to achieving and maintaining high standards of cleanliness and care for domestic and imported animals. The Department of Agriculture employs veterinarians to inspect livestock for diseases and to ensure humane conditions for farm animals in transit. The primary goal of the Public Health Service is protection: of animals against diseases and conversely, protection of humans who depend upon herd animals for food.

Veterinarians in the Department of Agriculture inspect meat and poultry, oversee quarantine procedures for imported animals and birds, and keep a vigilant eye on conditions in zoos, circuses and pet shops. It's reassuring to know that there is a

vast force of animal care professionals who see that animals—
meat-producing and exotic as well as companion—are
protected.

VETERINARY RESEARCH IN GOVERNMENT

Research offers many opportunities to the veterinarian-scien-
tist. The Department of Agriculture and the U.S. Public Health
Service have large divisions devoted to animal research. These
activities range from developing vaccines for the control of
animal ailments to the improvement of medicines to control
parasites.

VETERINARY RESEARCH IN INDUSTRY
AND MEDICINE

While the federal government conducts certain kinds of
research on behalf of animals and their producers, private
industry may have different research goals. Although many
companies are also looking for protective vaccines and exciting
new drugs, others may even involve the veterinarian in assuring
pets of good nutrition while pleasing their palates. Veterinar-
ian-researchers in one dog food company may study the reaction of test puppies to a new food. With hundreds of companies
marketing dog food, such canine test kitchens become deadly
serious weapons in the competitive battle for share-of-market.

An extremely valuable form of animal research is compara-
tive medicine, where veterinarians and medical doctors join
forces. With "firsts" in open heart surgery, spinal anesthesia
and similar new techniques to its credit, veterinary research is
understandably appreciated. Veterinarians and other animal
health professionals are also deeply involved in the animal

testing of new medical devices and procedures that precedes their approval by the Federal Drug Administration for human use.

A recent medical report that reflects today's advanced thinking in animal genetics (to name just one sub-specialty receiving attention) involves the work of a Pennsylvania veterinarian, Dr. Jonas Evans. Dr. Evans removes six- to eight-day-old embryos from the wombs of highly-bred, high-quality cows and implants them in the wombs of cows of lesser genetic quality. The result of this amazing and somewhat alarming-sounding procedure is that a dairy herd can be "upgraded" in a few years instead of 20 or more required with natural breeding. Meat is more tender, milk more abundant. The lower-quality surrogate birth-cow produces a high-bloodline calf—and the genetically superior cow is immediately freed to create another fetus of genetic superiority for implanting. In addition to domestic advantages, there are international implications; nutritionally-deprived countries with poorer-quality cows could produce better, more nutritious "products" with such an implant program in operation.

MILITARY VETERINARIANS

Veterinarians who serve in the armed forces may be involved in research, food inspection, animal sanitation and disease prevention. They may work in American military installations, or serve at U.S. bases overseas. Much of this work parallels the duties of a civilian veterinarian.

For instance, medical examinations of military watchdogs is similar to the work of the private small animal hospital. But one outstanding difference is that military animal practitioners may have to take helicopters to remote sites to reach their clients.

Joining the military means donning two uniforms: the military dress, and the doctor's whites. Military veterinarians feel a double sense of pride in serving their country and their profession.

ZOO VETERINARIAN

Chapter 10 is devoted to animal care careers centered on the modern zoo. But because many veterinarians opt for zoo careers full-time or serve as zoo consultants, their duties deserve a mention here.

Opportunities in zoos are limited for veterinarians because there are relatively few zoos. This is why many zoo veterinarians are consultants who devote a certain percentage of their practice time to zoo work in exchange for an agreed-upon yearly fee. The few full-time zoo veterinarians are very lucky to be in a specialty that combines the care of exotic animals with the role of animal preservationist and natural conservator.

Most zoo practice qualifies as "large animal" because of the diversity rather than the size of the animals in the veterinarians' care. But size is surely a factor. Witness the recent need of the Philadelphia Zoo's tiger, Monty, for a tooth extraction. Doctors and technicians at the University of Pennsylvania Veterinary Hospital handled the entire procedure from anesthetizing the 300-pounder to the removal of the abcessed tooth and the supervision of his post-op recovery. Specialists from anesthesiologist to veterinary surgeon were needed to do the job.

A typical day for a resident zoo veterinarian (or typical in-zoo activity for the part-time veterinary consultant) may include steps to control a disease unique to an important animal, an operation on a lion, and working with other zoo staffers in planning healthy, attractive new environments for the animals or advising on dietary needs and changes. These tasks are in addition to the regularly scheduled "rounds," those times when the veterinarian roams the zoo, observing all the birds, mammals and other creatures for signs of trouble.

As you can see, although the majority of veterinary students might logically select small animal practice, there are many fascinating options open to the graduating veterinarian.

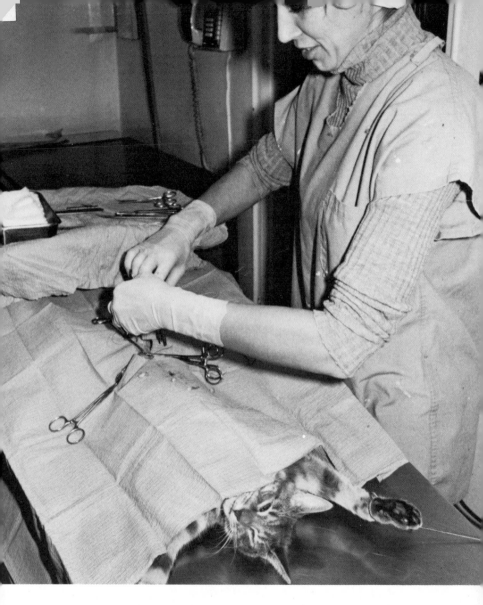

The job prospects for women in veterinary medicine are growing increasingly better. Photo: Ken Levinson.

CHAPTER 7

VETERINARY OUTLOOK FOR THE NEAR FUTURE

Many careers today are facing a period of instability. Career soothsayers hesitate to predict exactly how rosy or gloomy a field's future may be. Veterinary medicine is among the uncertain careers.

VETERINARY MEDICINE AND THE ECONOMY

Veterinary medicine was widely hailed in the early to mid-1970s as a career with unlimited potential with a projected shortage of 44,000 veterinarians by the early 1980s. The field now appears to be overcrowded.

Many things have happened since the '70s to affect the career outlook, recession and inflation among them. These developments forced families to trim their budgets for many things including proper pet care. Pet owners still think twice before they rush Friday or Gigi to the animal hospital for anything short of a dire emergency. These decisions to cut back on animal care spell revenue losses for veterinarians.

But pets and vets might be in for a happy surprise in the form of an insurance package that makes everybody happy. Veterinary Pet Insurance, for instance, is a program now offered by

700 California veterinarians. VPI offers accident protection for dogs and cats up to age 15 for $19 a year. Their major medical plan costs $44 to $109 a year, depending on the age of the insured pet. The maximum claim for a single procedure is $750. Surgery, dentistry and chemotherapy are among the items covered. If the concept spreads to other parts of the country, it could avoid the necessity of putting pets to sleep to avoid high medical expenses—and could mean added revenue for participating veterinarians.

IS THERE A SHORTAGE?

The shortage predictions of the '70s did not take place partly because more veterinary schools—27 instead of the 19 of the 1970s—have produced more graduates. These recent DVMs are now competing for clients with established veterinarians.

Arthur D. Little, Inc., a research organization, predicts an 8,300 surplus of veterinarians by the end of the decade. A recent American Veterinary Medicine Association report confirms the over-all slowdown in activity but does not provide statistics.

On a brighter note, the National Academy of Sciences predicts a 7% *increase* in the need for veterinarians in small, large and mixed animal practice in the next few years. Although this is a modest growth rate, it is a positive sign. And the Department of Labor, in a 1982-1983 publication, "Occupational Outlook Handbook," says that veterinary employment will *exceed* the average for other occupations through the 1980's. The Handbook cites tremendous interest in "companion" animals—the horse, the dog, and the cat—as reasons why the self-employed veterinarian will be able to make a successful living.

PROMISING FIELDS IN VETERINARY MEDICINE

The somewhat contradictory predictions for the self-employed practitioner do not reflect the whole field of veterinary medicine. Because the field is so diversified, there are areas where the employment outlook is quite healthy. Here are some examples.

DVM graduates who go on to earn degrees in toxicology (the science of poisons and their effects), parasitology (that area of biology dealing with organisms that thrive within living creatures), laboratory animal medicine and other specialties will find many jobs with corporations, in the public sector, and in veterinary military service. In addition, the veterinary field has expanded to include space medicine, international disease control and food production.

SOME OPTIMISM FOR PRIVATE PRACTICE

For those of you going to veterinary school because you want to build your own small or large animal practice, some optimism does exist. Mr. Michael Walters, Public Information Director of the American Veterinary Medical Association, says: "There will always be room for good veterinarians." With 40 million American families owning pets, this appears to be sound reasoning.

There are two promising developments within private veterinary practice. Continuing population growth makes the southwestern Sunbelt a good area for private practice at present. Also, veterinary practices specializing in large animals in rural areas are flourishing. Scientific methods for raising and breeding livestock and poultry are an increasing concern of the large animal practitioner. And the veterinarian who becomes involved in dairy production technology is pursuing a sure thing.

WOMEN IN VETERINARY MEDICINE

While veterinary medical career opportunities are somewhat uncertain, the outlook for women in the field is decidedly optimistic. Freshman classes in veterinary schools now reflect an almost even division of the sexes. Yet it was only a decade ago that a woman in this field was considered an oddity. High school guidance counselors discouraged girls from pursuing veterinary medicine as a career because of their supposed lack of physical strength and the difficulty of the work. But as the veterinary schools filled with women who began proving themselves on campus and later in practices, these fears of inadequacy diminished.

Where do women veterinarians choose to work? Most of them specialize in small animal medicine. A minority opt for a large animal specialty. But despite successful integration, women practitioners still encounter residual prejudice.

Dr. Ann Lucas, owner and director of the Washington Square Animal Hospital in Manhattan, tells of receiving middle-of-the-night emergency calls from panicked clients. Often when callers hear her voice, they ask to "speak to the veterinarian, please," assuming that she is an assistant. Dr. Lucas replies that she *is* the veterinarian, a fact they will have to accept if they want pre-dawn help.

SALARY EXPECTATIONS

Here are recent starting salary figures from the American Veterinary Medical Association.

Private Practice

Self-employed $18,400
Large animal 18,600
Mixed practice 17,200
Small animal 17,800

Other than private practice

College or university 13,000
Federal government 17,000
Armed forces 20,300
Industry 20,000
Other 18,600

Net income figures for experienced veterinarians:

Private practice

Large animal only $41,390
Predominantly large animal 39,015
Mixed animal 36,464
Small animal only 46,644
Predominantly small animal 38,333
Equine only 45,225

Other than private practice

College or university 32,043
Federal government 35,004
State and local government 30,254
Armed forces 26,814
Industry and other 43,185

Veterinarians in private practice can expect business-overhead and expenses to consume a considerable percentage of gross income. On the other hand, a thriving practice run by an enthusiastic, conscientious and businesslike practitioner will provide a comfortable living.

These figures are averages; those for beginners do not consider debt repayment for education. Income figures can also be considered to rise due to inflationary increases in the cost of animal health care, and in the general cost of living.

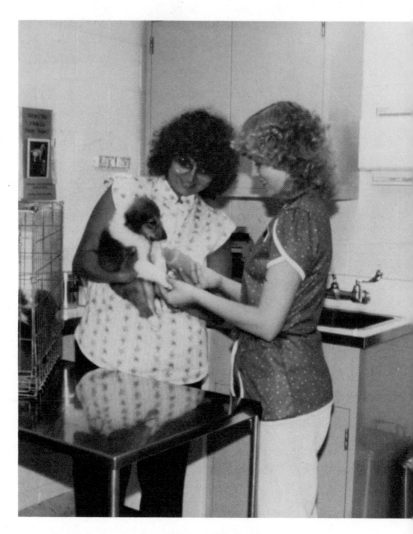

Working as a clerk in an animal hospital can be a good training experience. Photo: Michigan State University, College of Veterinary Medicine, Animal Technology Program and North American Veterinary Technicians Association.

CHAPTER 8

SUPPORT CAREERS FOR THE VETERINARY OFFICE: VETERINARY TECHNICIAN, ANIMAL LAB TECHNICIAN, ANIMAL HOSPITAL CLERK

The animal hospital has a strong "supporting cast" for veterinarians and their patients. These health care workers mentioned in the title may also be employed in animal shelters, in zoos and other animal care facilities.

THE VETERINARY TECHNICIAN

Animal care assistants may go under a variety of names—animal health technician, paraveterinarian, veterinary technician. Their responsibilities and duties generally coincide, varying only in the degree of responsibility assigned by the veterinarian.

One exception is the paraveterinarian or animal technologist with a Bachelor of Science (four-year) Degree in Veterinary Technology. He or she may *do* more and *earn* more than veterinary assistants graduating from a two-year animal technician program with an Associate in Applied Science or equivalent degree.

The position of animal health technician can be a happy compromise for you if for one reason or another you cannot become a veterinarian. Or, veterinary considerations aside, it is simply a rewarding job in a number of ways. Just think about the many areas in which these assistants may be involved: animal anesthesiology; surgical nursing; clinical conferencing; animal hospital management. Short of diagnosing, prescribing treatment and performing surgery, these animal care assistants can offer the animal patient the same comprehensive care as the veterinarian.

As mentioned in the Introduction, veterinary technicians have been hailed as indispensable team members in today's ultramodern intensive care units. Part nurse, part technician, they monitor an ill animal while offering it care and affection.

Student veterinary technicians graduating from any of the certified institutions in the country* have studied microbiology, radiology, animal husbandry, veterinary parasitology and other courses designed to give them a working knowledge of the veterinary field. While the curriculum sounds somewhat remote from the goal of animal and pet care, there is generally plenty of opportunity during the two-year study period to work with animals.

As a graduating animal technician, you can expect a starting salary ranging from $8,275 to $12,186. Experienced animal care assistants can earn from $8,407 to $16,016. (These are 1980 figures, the latest available at the time of writing; present salaries should be somewhat higher.) Openings are expected to increase throughout the 1980's because of the new, multi-purpose animal care centers with their sophisticated equipment.

---

* See the Appendix for a list of Animal Technician institutions.

So, the recently-graduated technician can look forward to a good job market and periodic advancement.

THE ANIMAL LAB TECHNICIAN

Of all the animal careers described in this book, animal laboratory technicians are the *least* involved with animals. Their work generally revolves around the prevention and treatment of animal diseases. Thus, test tubes and serums rather than animal care are their stock in trade.

But there is one role an animal lab technician or technologist may play that involves both experimentation and the animal world. The supervisor of a hospital or pharmaceutical animal laboratory constantly monitors a menagerie of mice, rats, dogs, rabbits and guinea pigs. Because these animals are there for research purposes, their environments must be carefully controlled and maintained to high standards, and their behavior must be constantly observed.

William Squires, supervisor of the Animal Laboratory of the Children's Hospital of Philadelphia, Pennsylvania, is responsible for the health of his laboratory animals. Each grouping of animals in the laboratory is separated from the others—rabbits from mice, for instance—so that each animal species is kept at its proper temperature and given its correct diet. Handling is also carefully controlled. Squires hold the animals gently but firmly so that the creatures sense that he is not frightened of them. (An animal sensing fear may try to bite the technician.)

A two-year Associate Degree in Applied Science has generally been acceptable for this field, but more and more aspiring technicians and technologists have been taking on four years of college. Science courses predominate in either a two- or four-year curriculum. Starting salaries range from $7,000 to $9,000 and may peak at $10,000 to $15,000 for the experienced animal

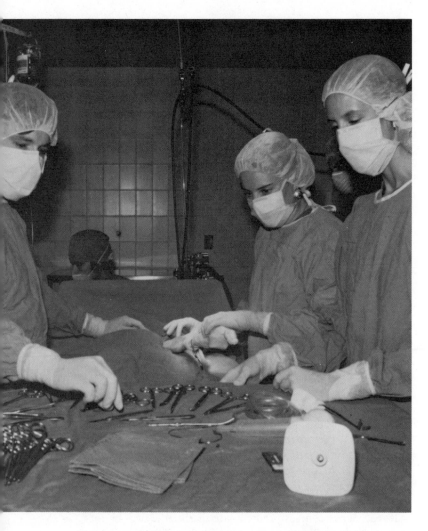
Veterinary technicians assist in surgery. Photo: University of Illinois College of Veterinary Medicine.

lab technician. Opportunities here are *abundant* according to the U.S. Government's Occupational Handbook.

THE ANIMAL HOSPITAL CLERK

The animal hospital clerk or receptionist is a familiar figure to the pet owner. This is the person who gathers up the trembling cat or dog and calls it soothingly by name. Because people view their pets as family members, they look for V.I.P. treatment from the minute they carry in their leashed, caged or boxed animals. That treatment begins at the front desk. The friendliness and competence of the animal hospital clerk are often the deciding factors in a pet owner's choice of a veterinary hospital or office.

Animal hospital clerks do far more than greet owner and pet. They have a multi-faceted job that may include record-keeping, billing, phone duty, making appointments, taking inventory, and expanding on the veterinarian's directions for treatment after the office visit—even to following-up by phone to see how the pet is doing.

An animal hospital clerk need not take courses beyond high school to qualify for this position. However, office skills and some knowledge of animals are helpful.

Starting salaries are in the range of $125 a week, and can rise to $150 or $165, depending on experience and the number of tasks expected.

Given the basic skills just outlined, a job as animal hospital clerk is an excellent beginning for the student desiring work while gaining further education in animal care or technology.

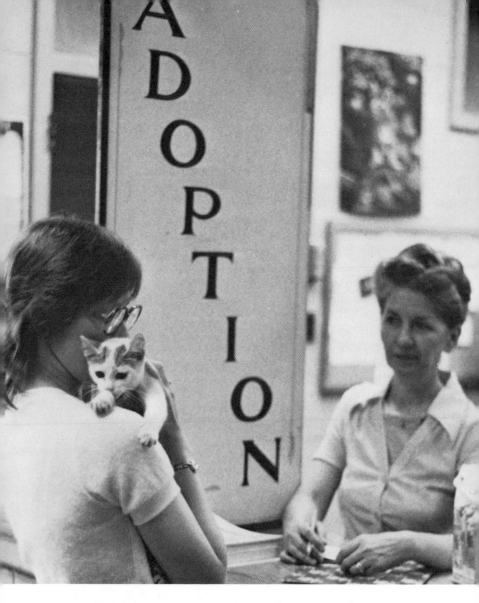

Animal shelters serve the community by acting as a source for pets.
Photo: Pennsylvania SPCA.

CHAPTER 9

PETS *IN* THERAPY AND
PETS *AS* THERAPY

While a dog can be one's best friend, it can also be a first-class nuisance. Barking dogs and yowling cats are not a joy to themselves or to others. Finally, someone is doing something about it. The pet psychologist (often called animal behaviorist) can help companion animals become pleasant members of their families. Therapy or re-training—often for as long as a year—is what it may take to make a pet a "civilized companion."

Conversely, pets are used in therapy to lessen the pain or loneliness of the sick, the handicapped and the elderly. Social workers and human psychologists are finding that the unconditional love pets can hold for people and their warm, furry presences can qualify them as effective members of the psychological treatment team.

Both these fields—pets in therapy and pets used as a part of therapy—are very recent, and are only now being recognized as fulfilling important needs. Some veterinary schools are ahead of others in introducing these areas into the curriculum.

MAKING THE PET A PLEASANT MEMBER
OF THE FAMILY

A barking, destructive, begging creature is not a household pet but a household *pest*. People will often put up with this obnoxious behavior just as they tolerate their own children's bad manners. Such disruption is unnecessary. Psychologists can analyze unacceptable animal behavior and in most cases can rectify it.

The University of Pennsylvania School of Veterinary Medicine initiated the Center for the Interaction of Animals and Society (with funding from the Geraldine R. Dodge Foundation). The Center, composed of researchers, veterinarians, animal behaviorists, psychologists, an anthropologist, several social workers and two psychiatrists, seeks better understanding of the interaction between animals and humans.

One of the animal behaviorists, Dr. Victoria Voith, has chosen to concentrate on the behavior of the aggressive, unsociable pet. One client was an owner afraid to return home at night to her belligerent Doberman Pinscher. The cure for the unfriendly Doberman was to show it who was boss. Since the dog had taken the authority role as his own, there was a lot of relearning to do. This repatterning consisted of teaching the dog to become dependent upon his owner. His mistress taught the dog to sit or lie down before he was fed or walked. Gradually, the animal got the point, and the proper household balance was restored. Another client's dog left a trail of broken furniture behind as he tried to "escape" a thunder and lightning storm.

Dr. Voith does not make house calls; the animal and owner come to the Veterinary School for $25-per-hour office visits. Sessions last from one to three hours, and then the owner and pet depart with "homework" instructions.

A New York psychologist, Dr. Donald Tortora, has just become coordinator of an animal behavior-therapy clinic in

Manhattan. His fees—matching the city's inflated costs—are $45 an hour to "modify" animal behavior. One of the animal psychologist's recent cases involved a problem almost universally shared by dog owners: pets rearrange the furniture when left alone for long periods. Translated, "rearranging" means they break, upend or nudge chairs, tables, even sofas, from their normal places.

In most cases, the dog is misbehaving because he or she is upset or even bored at being left alone. One solution is to have the owners go out and return frequently in the first few days of training, so that the stay-at-home learns that he won't be left alone for long.

Because it is the animal's "psychology" to react to something the owner is doing—in this case, returning home more frequently—he will gradually let up on the destruction. The cause of his loneliness is perceived as being lessened, so he doesn't need to carry on. Once this behavior modification has taken place, the owners may again leave for increasingly longer periods because the retraining has been successful.

A NEW CAREER: THERAPY—PETS FOR THE SICK, ELDERLY AND HANDICAPPED

While companion animals may need a man-to-dog talk every so often to correct unattractive habits, they can in turn prove to be of immeasurable help in solving human-based problems.

Consider this: the attention pets give humans is known to help regulate heartbeat, lower blood pressure and calm nerves. People with animals tend to live longer and are sick less frequently. They are less tense because the animal's bids for attention interrupt stressful activity whether related to home or work. If animals can do this for ordinary, healthy people, think what positive effects they could have on the sick, handicapped or elderly! Although people have recognized the therapeutic effects of their dogs and cats for centuries, they have only recently applied the knowledge in a scientific way—and a new animal career is born.

What is so special about a pet? Dogs in particular give unstintingly of their love while expecting nothing in return. They will pour out affection on demand and provide a soothing kind of companionship. Cats, while often more independent, are also comforting, and their furriness and warmth are a source of pleasure.

Eleanor L. Ryder, a former zoologist and now a professor at the School of Social Work of the University of Pennsylvania, works closely with the University's School of Veterinary Medicine. Her most recent interest involves pets and the elderly. These are not the senior citizens of retirement communities and nursing homes but those who are living active, independent lives.

Most thrive on the affection of their pets, Ms. Ryder finds, and are more alert because of them. The social worker is also interested in the types and breeds of pets most suitable for older people.

While Ms. Ryder studies the benefits of pets for the independent elderly, recreational therapists at the Veterans Administration Center in Salem, Virginia, bring companion animals to visit the oldsters who call this facility "home." This very special program of animal visitation is a weekly planned project, and the reaction of the residents to the pets is astonishing. Many, initially slumped in wheelchairs, heads nodding, become alert and animated by the arrival of a gaggle of small animals, brought courtesy of the local SPCA.

The pets dissipate loneliness, encourage alertness and stimulate under-used minds. As Ms. Susan Jones, head of the pet-people program, says, "The program gives the staff something to do with patients besides taking their temperatures."

Animals also offer the same special qualities to the sick and handicapped. They can be particularly helpful to the seriously ill child. A recent and touching case of an "extended paw" involved a 12-year-old English girl and her mongrel pet, Robbie. Doctors credited the improvement of Alison Hart of Bournemouth, England, to the large, friendly dog. Alison, often depressed about her debilitating kidney disease, was coaxed out of her gloom by Robbie's insistent but loving demand for her attention.

VETERINARY SOCIAL WORKERS HELP PET OWNERS COPE WITH ILLNESS, DEATH

There is yet another guidance area for the pet psychologist or animal social worker, but in this case, the therapy largely involves the pet owner.

Psychologists now realize that owners who must consider euthanasia—the merciful putting-to-sleep—of very old or hopelessly ill animals, or those who have just had their animals euthanized are in an emotional turmoil. These professionals are easing the suffering of the pet owner by acknowledging the pain and loneliness they feel, and by helping them to express their grief and by this process, to recover from it.

Jamie Quackenbush, a veterinary social worker, bridges the two disciplines needed for this work. He is a doctoral candidate at the University of Pennsylvania School of Social Work as well as being a research associate in the University's Veterinary Hospital. Mr. Quackenbush helps people cope with the death of a pet. He knows that, for some, the loss of a beloved animal can trigger abnormal depression—even thoughts of suicide. But for those fortunate enough to talk with him, recovery usually proceeds normally. Quackenbush tells owners referred to him that such depression after a pet's death is normal. He encourages

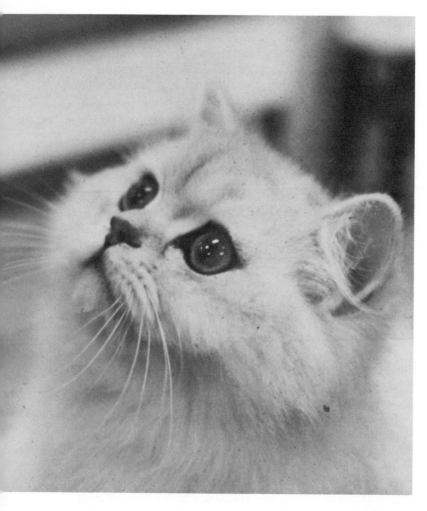

Animals can elicit affection from all sorts of people. Photo: Michigan State University, College of Veterinary Medicine, Animal Technology Program and North American Veterinary Technicians Association.

their expressions of grief and responds with consolation. "I understand. Things are quite different for you. You feel anger and pain—but do remember all the happy times you had with your pet."

This emotional aid extends beyond the time of the animal's death. Mr. Quackenbush may talk with the owner several times in the first week, even into the weeks that follow if there is still difficulty in adjusting to the loss.

This veterinary social worker's activities are not limited to "animal bereavement," the formal title for his work. Mr. Quackenbush is also available to help an owner through the anxious periods of a pet's major illness or operation. If an owner is too unstrung to go through hospital formalities when admitting a pet, Jamie Quackenbush will fill out forms, carry the pet's blanket and do whatever else will make the situation a bit less painful for the owner. He will also explain the testing or operation procedures, and how fully the doctors predict recovery, and help the owner achieve a more positive frame of mind.

Thus, pets are helpers for humans, and in turn, they are helped by caring people. This mutual dependence is as it should be, because each has so much to give the other.

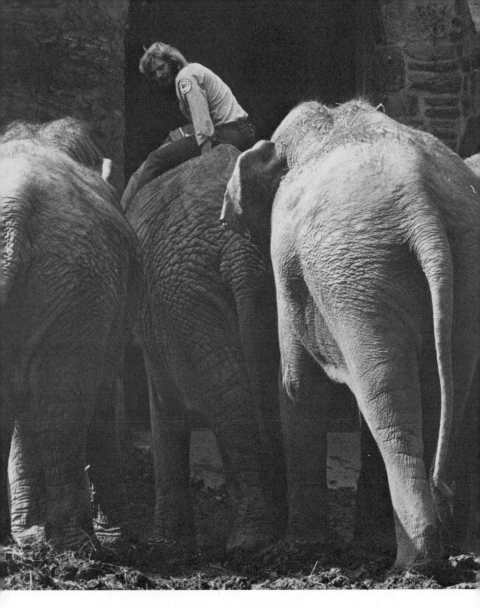

Dave Wood of the Zoological Society of Philadelphia is the zoo's elephant keeper. Photo: Zoological Society of Philadelphia.

CHAPTER 10

VARIETY AND EXCITEMENT IN ZOO WORK AND WILD ANIMAL TRAINING

SOME ZOO CAREERS

Classified ads may list jobs from A to Z, but "zoo" is rarely among them. Zoo careers are far from the "top ten" job opportunities for the 1980's. Yet, jobs are there, many of them avenues to advancement.

What makes up the zoo "family" (animals excluded)? Large zoos have a director, resident or visiting veterinarian, habitat designer, curators and a photographer who may double as director of public relations. The backbone workers, of course, are the zoo keepers. Smaller zoos hire fewer people, and everyone does multiple jobs. Large or small, the zoo staff pulls together to put on a "show" almost 365 days a year—the showing of its fascinating residents to the public.

ZOO DIRECTOR

Zoo directors may have come up through the ranks, their experience as zoo keepers and curators making them ideal candidates for directorships. Or their job entry may be through a Degree in Zoology, a background in animal management, or because of the letters "D.V.M." after their names. Whatever their field of expertise, zoo directors often have advanced degrees plus experience in business administration, an understanding of animals' natural habitats, and a dedication to animal conservation.

The director has to orchestrate the different activities of the zoo: animal nutrition; budget concerns; the purchase of animals; the creation of naturalistic displays—and everything to do with personnel.

In community and county zoos, the director may have similar duties, but would serve as well as curator, librarian—even zoo keeper—when the occasion warrants.

Salaries vary widely, depending on the largesse of the zoo's city or town. Salaries may range from $10,000 to $40,000 in these hard-to-come-by jobs.

ZOO CURATOR

Zoo curators are in charge of the various zoological units. While there may be only one curator in charge of all animals in a small zoo, large zoos have curators who are specialists in one area: birds; mammals; reptiles and perhaps fishes.

Each curator oversees the buildings which are the animals' homes, creating a comfortable environment that also displays each animal to advantage. As curators go through their daily routine, they may meet a hundred challenges, from an unexpected animal ailment to signs of a hoped-for birth, or the carefully controlled shifting of animals from one cage to another.

Here's the profile of a young lady who is eminently qualified for her position. Chris Shepard, a Californian, is presently curator of birds at the Bronx Zoo in New York. Years of study preceded her entry into the world of the zoo. Chris received a Ph.D. in Ecology and Evolutionary Biology before she put her academics to work in her career with birds, her favorite subject. Fortunately for Chris, there was a curator-training program available at the Bronx Zoo. From this internship, she stepped into the role of curator of birds.

Her charges number into the hundreds—brightly feathered, exotic birds that take over a several-stories-tall building. Many are there because Chris selected them. When she chooses her species, she considers compatibility with other birds, and breeding potential. Endangered birds, or those with diminishing populations earn extra attention from Chris—increasing their population is a real challenge.

Beginning curators like Chris Shepard can earn $10,000 to start, and in a well-endowed zoo, can advance to $20,000—$30,000 as they gain experience.

Curators generally have advanced degrees in Zoology or a related area, and have had some previous experience in zoo park management or zoo-keeping.

ZOO KEEPER

Zoo keepers are primarily responsible for the *direct* care and feeding of the animals in a particular "house." Whether the lion, bird, monkey or reptile house, as a zoo keeper, you would have intimate, daily contact with these animal residents. Cages must be cleaned and hosed or swept (the occupants are usually moved to another cage while this is done) and the animals given fresh water and their allotment of food.

But zoo animal keepers are far more than housemaids. They are also *nurse*maids—or at least keen observers of their animals' well-being. Should a monkey, crocodile or kangaroo show signs of illness, the zoo keeper as trained observer reports any symptoms to the veterinarian, the curator, or others responsible for an animal's condition.

A zoo keeper may also be an expert on animal breeding, be familiar with the irregular habits of rare species, and be capable of arranging animal habitats and assisting with exhibit planning and building.

Mothering—or fathering—may be another duty of the zoo keeper. Often, animal-infants are raised in a nursery away from the parent. The animal mother may *not* "mother," ignoring or rejecting her offspring, as she sees fit. Or the litter may be so large that a small creature might lose out on the mother's love and nourishment. In this case, the keeper becomes surrogate parent, feeding, rocking or playing with the baby animal.

Later, when the animal is ready, the keeper may reestablish the youngster in the family setting. The keeper does this with a watchful eye—and often, a prayer. Some animals simply do not get a happy reception, and are summarily rejected by parent or siblings.

Animal education (zoology or animal husbandry) or extensive work with animals are prerequisites for the job of zoo keeper. Assistant zoo keepers begin at the low end of the scale—in the $5,000 range, but as they rise, they can pass the $10,000 a year mark. Head zoo keepers can earn up to $18,000.

WILD ANIMAL TRAINER

While zoo careers offer close contact with animals, they do not bring you as close to members of the Animal Kingdom— literally!—as wild animal training.

To succeed in this field, you need two very different characteristics: an empathy or kinship with wild animals, and the courage and agility to face and deal with them. You will also need long and extremely thorough training. Most animal trainers say their *own* training never ends, nor does that of their animals.

There are several large circuses and quite a few smaller ones where you could work if you have the necessary skills. Some thirty circuses still exist, along with another hundred or so smaller traveling shows that entertain in shopping malls, at state and county fairs and similar "grandstand" locations. There are also safari parks near major cities where animals perform, as well as some zoos that offer animal acts, and "sea-quarium" attractions with their showoff seals and sea lions.

The animal trainer is basically a performer, tuned-in to the cheers of the crowd and willing to accept the often difficult conditions of seasonal travel—constant movement, long hours, less than luxurious surroundings. As an animal trainer, you are "show biz," putting on one or more shows a day, and spending long hours in between caring for your animals and ever-improving your act. A large part of your eventual success as a personality will come from the creativeness of your act—the exciting combination of daring, showmanship and originality.

Make no mistake, animal training is a hazardous way to earn a living. The two basic rules are: one, be aware 60 seconds of every minute of the moods of your animals (and know that they have a "sixth sense" for *your* moods); two, never allow yourself to get in a situation where you have to trust a wild animal even for a moment.

Part of the thrill for an audience is the very real danger in which the trainer works. Whips, chairs and guns that fire blanks aren't used by trainers for show, but serve to distract an animal and keep it in line when the trainer senses it is about to do something that's *not* on the program!

There is no school for animal trainers except the real world of experience. Even a youngster whose parents are animal trainers starts learning just where the outsider does, at the beginning.

That "beginning" can come while you are still in high school, provided you are able to find summer work with a traveling show or at a safari park. At the start, it will probably not be with animals; the idea is to get a job doing whatever is available from selling popcorn to taking tickets. Once you are in, be persistent about working with animals and maybe you'll get a lucky break. You might feed the beasts or clean their cages. It will at least prove your ability to move around animals, and will certainly help you to understand them.

Whether or not you work with animals at first, take all the time you legitimately can to watch the trainers at work. This is definitely a learning-by-doing career, but it must be preceded with a long period of learning-by-watching.

If your luck holds, you will become apprenticed to a trainer, and will later serve as an assistant. Your involvement will, of course, be the dirty work: loading and unloading the animals, feeding them, and keeping them and their environment clean and healthy.

Feeding is the key to your early instruction in wild animal training, because all training works on a reward system. A leopard can be trained to hop on a stool if meat is placed on it. And other animals can be taught to perform, provided the reward appears on schedule. If you as the trainer are always the person associated with the reward, you are the one for whom the animals will perform.

If this sounds easy, it isn't. Some animal trainers say it takes up to two years of constant work to create a good animal act, perhaps twice that time to make the act exceptional.

One of the duties you will perform before you can begin to work with animals is assisting the trainer as part of your apprenticeship. Among other things, you will be called upon to watch the trainer's act. You will observe all the animals all the time, to see things the trainer cannot: what the animals *not* under the trainer's direct control are doing, or thinking of doing. To do this job well will take weeks, even months, of careful observing and understanding of each animal's nature and temperament. You would, of course, observe from outside the training cage and warn the trainer of anything that might seem to be going wrong.

In training, your approach to the animals should be extremely patient, as though you were training a very young child. The keys are constant repetition of each command with its necessary action such as tickling or prodding the animal, always followed by praise and reward. Animals can also be taught what you do *not* want them to do, by adroit use of a prod, whip, or even slaps to discourage misbehavior. This is a form of instruction in the hands of a skilled trainer—never carried to the degree where it verges on cruelty or causes the animal to attack.

Working with more than one animal or more than one type at a time is a necessary part of developing an animal act. This calls for a long period of getting the different animals used to each other. To start with, tigers and lions, for instance, are caged next to each other, then "introduced" in the same cage but controlled with collars and chains. The trainer gets them to look forward to this mingling by giving them meat as a reward. Gradually, the animals are worked with longer chains as they accept the presence of the trainer. The collars and chains are removed as the actual training progresses. Patience, kindness, vigilance and courage are essential during every second of the process—in fact, during every second the trainer works or performs with animals.

In addition to lions, tigers and elephants—the most popular animals—monkeys, bears, kangaroos and sea lions rate high with audiences. Training of dogs and horses as performers also calls for patience and stamina, but does not involve the high risks of wild animal training.

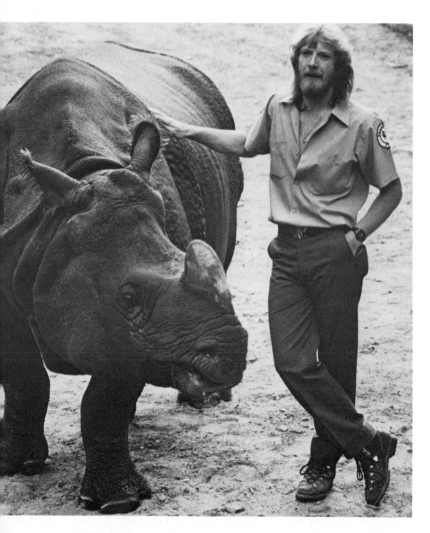

Wild animals in captivity require special care. Photo: Zoological Society of Philadelphia.

The trainer may well have a long day—especially if he or she is touring (which usually means rocky sleep until you get used to it). The animals must be fed twice a day, cleaning must be done, costumes and props readied, rehearsals and more training carried out, and one or more shows performed. Life is a bit easier—but not much—for animal trainers who work in safari parks and other non-touring attractions. Should an animal get sick, that, too, becomes the trainer's responsibility.

After a suitable paid apprenticeship with at least one trainer but often with more (to gain varied experience), most trainers go out on their own just as any theatrical performer does. He or she usually owns the animals they perform with, once they establish their act. The pay for independent trainers varies according to their skills and reputations. A top-rated act may pay very well; a relative beginner might be lucky to break even. In addition to the cost of the animals, ongoing expenses include food, medical care, costumes, props and pay for an assistant or apprentice. Should the trainer be injured—a not unlikely possibility—the costs go on even if the act does not. The ever-present personal danger is the greatest drawback to this profession—one reason why it is relatively uncrowded.

As for opportunities, they do exist, although the American circus is no longer "in the center ring" of entertainment. As we have seen, many circuses still tour "under canvas." In addition to the stationary amusement centers mentioned, there are also opportunities in training animals for use in TV shows and motion pictures. The *Star Wars* creature, Bantha, was really an outrageously costumed elephant, and the "actor" who rode between its giant curved horns was its trainer, Bob Spiker.

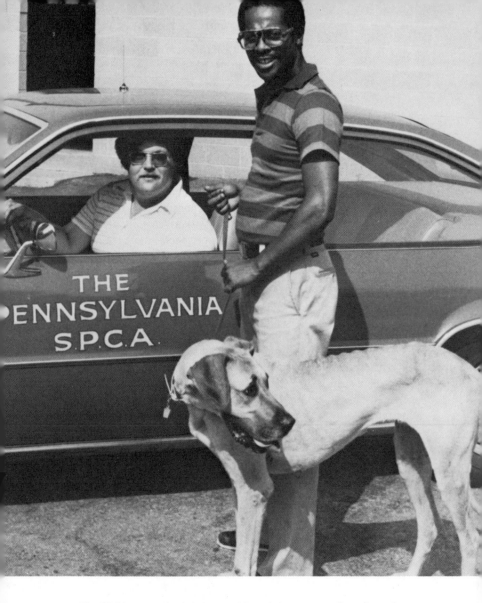

The SPCA runs animal shelters and investigates reports of cruelty and neglect. Photo: Pennsylvania SPCA.

CHAPTER 11

CAREERS IN ANIMAL SHELTERS AND PET SHOPS

Although they are quite different, these two areas are covered together because both offer excellent job (or volunteer) opportunities for beginners in animal care. With experience, you can advance in either area, or use that experience as a stepping stone to a different animal care career.

ANIMAL SHELTER CAREERS

With a high school diploma—or during summer vacations—you can enter animal shelter work with a paid or volunteer job as a kennel worker or adoption clerk. With a diploma and perhaps some additional schooling you can apply for a job as an Animal Control Officer (also called Humane Agent). With further education and training, you can rise through the organization to become an Animal Control Supervisor, Assistant Shelter Manager, Shelter Manager, Humane Education Specialist, or to the top post in the animal shelter, Executive Director (also called Director of Animal Control).

To understand why some jobs have two titles, you should know about the two types of animal shelters. And to see how well you might fit into the picture, you need to know the characteristics that all animal shelter workers have in common.

ANIMAL SHELTER TYPES

There are two kinds of animal shelters. Some 550 are operated by SPCAs and humane societies, often in cooperation with local government, which assists with funding and law enforcement. They are run by Executive Directors and their outside animal workers are called Humane Agents. These shelters depend largely on contributions.

Approximately 2,000 other shelters are supported by their cities and towns. Their leaders are usually called Directors of Animal Control, and their outside workers are known as Animal Control Officers. Many of these agencies perform their own law enforcement.

ANIMAL SHELTER FUNCTIONS

Both shelters do the same things for the communities:
- Enforce local animal control and licensing laws
- Investigate complaints of cruelty or animal nuisances
- Issue citations against lawbreakers and testify in court against them
- Control stray, injured, or unwanted animals
- Rescue animals
- Inspect animal facilities for compliance with laws
- Care for animals in their custody
- Find new homes for animals through adoption
- Put animals to sleep that cannot be adopted

With all these jobs to be done, there is much work available for the animal shelter employee or volunteer.

CHARACTERISTICS NEEDED FOR
ANIMAL SHELTER WORK

Some people who have selected animal care careers say it's because they relate better to animals than to people. The animal shelter worker should be an exception, since a large part of any job from Director to adoption clerk involves a high degree of public contact and calls for good public relations. Shelter workers must deal positively with the public while dealing kindly with the animals that are their prime responsibility.

Part of this public relations involves the often difficult task of making people aware of the animal shelter's mission, which is community service. The old stereotype of the shelter as being merely "the dog pound" unfortunately persists. Although enforcing local dog laws is still one duty, shelter workers' jobs go far beyond that old-fashioned notion.

Positive public relations is also needed to overcome the negative perception of euthanasia—an unfortunate necessity in the face of animal abandonment and pet over-population.

Much animal shelter work could be heartbreaking for the people doing it. A high proportion of the animals the worker deals with are not suitable for adoption and must be destroyed. Even with a well-publicized adoption program, the supply of pets often exceeds the demand. Shelter workers' natural compassion must be tempered with professionalism in the face of reality if they are to serve the community's need for animal control.

Another necessary characteristic is the willingness to work for relatively low pay, particularly in animal shelters funded by public contributions. In many areas, the funds for shelter operation are barely adequate, and pay is proportionately less than it might be for work at similar levels in other animal care areas.

SHELTER JOBS FOR BEGINNERS

The *kennel worker* is one of the animal shelter mainstays. This job can lead to promotion within the shelter, or to a job as *Control Officer* or *Humane Agent*. If you think that animal shelter work is your cup of kibble but you have no experience, a summer of paid work or volunteering will give you an insider's perspective on things. As a kennel worker, you will care for sick and well animals in separate areas, feed puppies, dogs, kittens, cats and other creatures, keep them and their cages clean, and perhaps help with adoptions and learn to do some administrative detail. If you are not a volunteer, you will very likely be paid close to minimum wage for your efforts, but you'll acquire that all-important experience in animal care that will be invaluable in any animal care career you select. As a volunteer, especially if you are in college with an animal-related major, you may be able to get some sort of course credit for your summer internship, a possibility well worth investigating ahead of job time.

The *shelter adoption clerk* helps people select the right pets (or reclaim their lost animals), completes the adoption papers, collects the necessary fees, and instructs the new owners in basic pet care. This, too, can be either a full-time job or an internship. A pleasing personality, affinity for animals, basic typing, administrative and telephone skills and a high school diploma are the usual requirements. As with kennel worker, the opportunity for experience or possible advancement should be more important to you than earnings.

ANIMAL CONTROL OFFICER/HUMANE AGENT

Regardless of the name, this is the high-visibility animal shelter job. In the city-operated shelter, Animal Control Officer is the usual title; Humane Agent is the name for the same job in the SPCA or humane society facility. This is the person most often viewed by the public—positively or negatively depending on whether the job at hand is rescuing a kitten for a grateful child or filing a cruelty complaint against the irate owner of a roadside zoo.

This is a job you may be able to get if you're a high school graduate with good communication skills, a positive (but not overbearing) manner and the ability to make sound judgments on the spot. A background in basic law enforcement, animal science or veterinary technology is helpful but may not be essential. In several states, your proficiency in animal law enforcement has to be legally certified, often as a part of your on-the-job training.

Physically, this job calls for skill in animal handling and control (again, part of training), stamina, agility, and a degree of strength. Pure strength is not as important as gentleness and persuasiveness. For this reason, women make excellent Officers, and many are entering the field.

As a new Officer, you would first have several weeks of training in animal law, recognition of animal breeds and behavior, illnesses, injuries and symptoms of disease. In the next training period, you would learn the animal capture and handling techniques for all the situations you'd be likely to encounter. You'd also receive training in dealing with the public.

After you begin work—often as a partner with an experienced Officer—it usually takes two months or more for you to become reasonably competent. As a beginner, you might be the vehicle driver, assisting and learning from your partner as you make daily rounds.

Your control team may start the day with a list of requests and complaints to be checked out: a barking dog; a roving monkey; a treed cat. Other requests may come in by two-way radio: a pig has escaped from an overturned truck on the Interstate, or a skunk needs to removed from a suburban garage.

As you rescue, capture or administer first aid, your team would try to find the owners of domestic animals, and might issue a warning or write a citation for an unlicensed animal. Only when animals are wild, injured or without apparent owners are they taken to the shelter.

Officers most often find the public is cooperative. In the rare instance when a pet owner becomes troublesome or a situation gets out of hand—when your one escaped pig turns out to be a squealing herd—your team would call for shelter or police reinforcements by radio. In any event, an Officer's day is seldom dull.

One such Spring day was exciting indeed for Janie Gerber, head Control Officer of the Aspen/Pitkin County (Colorado) Animal Control Department. Responding to a call, she found a kitten marooned on a rock in a river, trapped by rising flood waters. Janie called for volunteers from the many spectators, formed a human chain, and plunged into the raging water to rescue the kitten. She succeeded, and took the kitten to a local veterinarian even before changing her soaked clothing.

Janie Gerber, an avid outdoorsperson, performs human rescue work in Colorado's rugged mountains during the winter snows. She has trained her own German Shepherd to help.

Janie is also deeply involved in humane education, and is a favorite speaker at area service clubs and Scout meetings. She believes that the more people know about the needs of animals, the more responsive—and responsible—they will be.

In some areas, you, like Janie, would aid in public relations by speaking on pet care and shelter operation to civic and school groups. You would also make inspection and enforcement calls on pet shops, zoos, animal processing centers, traveling circuses or shows and riding stables, either at random or in answer to complaints. When rounds are over, you would enter reports on the animals brought in, the citations issued, and the findings of your inspections.

Full-time work is usually found only in areas with populations of 100,000 or more. In smaller communities and rural areas, Agents or Officers often work part-time and hold other jobs. Part-time salaries are from $3,000 to $8,000 a year; full-time beginners earn from $7,500 to $12,000 a year. Senior Officers or Agents in larger communities can earn $16,000 or more a year.

HUMANE EDUCATION SPECIALIST

With additional schooling beyond high school, your chances for interesting shelter career work grow. Among the jobs available are veterinary technician (see Chapter 8) and humane education specialist. Higher education is the key to shelter management positions as well.

Humane education specialist is a relatively new career with moderate growth. If you elect to enter it, be prepared to get a college degree in elementary education first, with a minor in animal science of biology. You should also plan to live in a major population area, since most humane education specialists work for larger humane societies, often in connection with an area's public school system.

Your job would be educating the public—especially school children—on the need for humane treatment and respect for animals. Your tasks would very likely include conducting audio-visual lectures, field trips, pet care classes and wildlife preservation courses. You might also be the public relations liaison between your humane society and the community.

Salaries for humane education specialists range from about $8,000 to $16,000, depending on qualifications, experience and the size of the community you would serve. The Humane Society of the United States (HSUS) can provide more information about this career specialty.

ANIMAL SHELTER MANAGEMENT CAREERS

The top management position in the humane society shelter is *Executive Director;* the same person in the city-connected facility is the Director of Animal Control. In either shelter, the second in command is called the Shelter Manager. In smaller facilities, these jobs may be combined.

The Director is like the captain of a ship—in charge of every phase of the operation. He or she must have excellent administrative, personnel management and public relations skills. In a municipal facility, the Director formulates the annual budget, in cooperation with a City Council or other governing group, then operates the facility within the budget. The Director may also be expected to raise money if the center operates on a contract that does not cover all its expenses.

The Executive Director of a humane facility usually works with a Board of Directors, and is an unofficial member. The Executive Director is also the chief fundraiser, an important job—and in either facility, the Director maintains harmonious relations with the public, by appearing often on local radio and TV talk shows, and by seeking favorable publicity for the shelter's programs and operations.

Although Directors may rise through the ranks—most often promoted from Shelter Managers—they may also have had experience as veterinarians, commercial kennel operators, or animal science specialists. Directors can earn from $12,000 to $20,000 depending on the type, size and location of the animal shelter. Salaries for Directors in large cities can range up to $40,000 a year. Since Directorship openings are relatively rare, an aspiring Director must be willing to relocate when and where an opening appears.

In shelters large enough to need them, the Director is aided by a *Shelter Manager,* in charge of all day-to-day activities from supervising employees to maintaining cleanliness standards and purchasing supplies. The careers leading to Manager are similar to Director, including advancement from within. Salaries are slightly below those for Directors, from $12,000 to $20,000, perhaps $30,000 if the Manager also functions as Director.

At both top management levels, a thorough knowledge of animal health standards, community expectations and animal law enforcement are required for the job.

Middle management jobs offer salaries higher than Control Officer but below Shelter Manager. These can include Control Officer Supervisor (or Humane Agent Supervisor) and Assistant Shelter Manager. These jobs are usually earned through promotion, or by changing from one animal shelter to another.

ANIMAL CONTROL WORKSHOPS

If you are fortunate enough to live in or near certain major population areas, you could learn a great deal about animal welfare and animal control by attending an animal control workshop. The locations are:

- HSUS workshops—minimum of four two-day workshops are held yearly in different sections of the country, often as part of state humane society business meetings.

- Virginia Polytechnic Institute workshops—three six-session workshops a year.
- Texas A&M workshop—a five-day short course in Animal Personnel Training.
- Massachusetts SPCA Humane Agent Training Program—an eight-week formal training course.

More about these courses can be found in "Careers: Working with Animals—the Humane Society's Guide" by Guy Hodge, published by the Humane Society of the United States, 2100 L Street N.W., Washington, DC 20037.

PET SHOP CAREERS

Although they are at the other end of the pet care spectrum from animal shelters, pet shops also offer work for beginners. Summer or after-school work in a pet shop can give you the edge in experience that can help you enter another area of animal care—or can help you develop the selling and management skills you'll need to operate a pet-related business of your own.

Some pet stores sell both common and exotic animals, and offer supplies and grooming services as well (this is an excellent separate business, too). Other shops stick to the basics: kittens, puppies, gerbils, hamsters and fish. Some merchants specialize in fish or birds—and if the shop is called Jim's Puppyland, you know what to expect when you walk in. But whatever the merchandising philosophy, the job skills for beginners are the same: willingness, love of animals, a sense of order and cleanliness, and an ability to deal with people.

Pet store work often begins early. The pets may be fed before the doors open for business. Cage cleaning goes on until all are fresh. Animals are inspected for illness and—surprise!—unexpected pregnancies. Customers select pets and supplies, new animals are checked and added to waiting cages, pet supply salesmen are welcomed (they are a top source of merchandising ideas, many pet shop owners say). On days when the store is closed, the pets must still be fed, watered, and their cages kept clean. Most of these are jobs you as a beginner can do.

With experience, and ongoing education into how to run a retail business, you can advance in the pet shop world, perhaps to manager of a store, or to the ownership of your own shop.

If you do go into business for yourself, take the advice of experienced pet shop owners and locate your store in a high traffic area. It's not surprising that many pet stores are in shopping malls where people can stroll in comfort regardless of the weather, and where children predominate in the crowds that pass by. Learn to plan appealing window displays; many pets and supplies are bought on irresistible impulse, and the sight of your appealing window will draw customers inside.

While minimum wage is generally the rule for pet shop workers who are also students, you may receive modest pay increases the longer you stick with the job, and the more willing you are to do the dirty chores. Or, your boss may let you work behind the counter and add a small sales commission to your hourly wages. Later, as your own boss, it is possible to earn $20,000 or more a year over and above your shop's expenses.

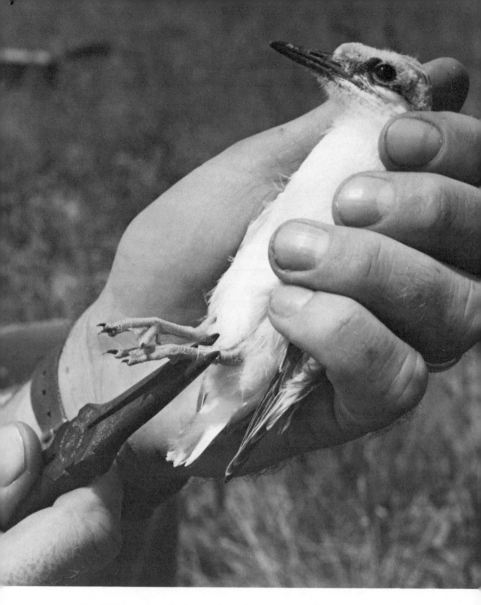

A wildlife conservationist bands the leg of a young Least Tern. Photo: Jack P. Dermid, Bureau of Sport Fisheries and Wildlife.

CHAPTER 12

CAREERS IN ANIMAL WILDLIFE, CONSERVATION, AND COMMUNICATIONS

THE CONSERVATION ATTITUDE

Remember in Chapter 2 we mentioned the "commodity" attitude toward wildlife that prevailed in America until the turn of the century?

This attitude, that wild animals and the wilderness itself are there for people's use and are not of value for themselves, still exists, a holdover from the days when most of this country was uncharted wilderness and land and animals were ours for the taking. The degree to which this attitude continues is in part political, but not necessarily pervasive in the government-run parks and forests. As national administrations change, the protectionist-versus-commodity controversy swings with it. As this is written, the commodity end of the seesaw is carrying more weight than in previous administrations. As you read this, however, continuing pressure exerted by conservation groups may once more be advancing environmental causes, to the improvement of the presently static job market.

Most animal wildlife careers are government-funded, either by the federal government or by the individual states. While that funding may fluctuate—and job possibilities with it—the basic course is still in the direction established by landmark groups such as the Sierra Club (founded in 1892) and by later arrivals on the conservation scene: that the need to maintain America's open lands and preserve our native wildlife is essential to the country's ecological future. With the slow but steady acceptance of this perspective, career opportunities will continue to expand, as will work with conservation organizations. But be warned—this expansion is neither strong nor immediate.

BASIC CAREER REQUIREMENTS

Wildlife and conservation work calls for strong mathematical and communications skills. Endurance and a duck's ability to shed water are handy, too, because much of the work is done outdoors often under difficult conditions. Self-reliance is another good trait to have, since counting the tracks of animals that appear in response to attractive scent—one method of surveying their numbers—may call for many days of observation alone in deep woods.

Workers in national and state parks may be involved in both animal and people management, one place where communications enters the picture. Also, animal technicians who manage wildlife and land resources must be skilled statistical analysts and reporters, able to chart and interpret changes in migration and feeding patterns and animal populations.

Your duties might include the banding of wild animals and birds, conducting wildlife and ecological surveys, animal population regulation, the preservation or development of natural habitats to help in animal propagation, experimentation with bird and animal food sources, and the protection and rescue of animals from natural or manmade disasters.

Other duties include the enforcement of fishing, hunting and camping laws, park direction, communication and public relations.

Wildlife technicians work for a variety of agencies including industry, state fish and game commissions, privately-funded wildlife preserves, and conservation organizations. The largest single employer, however, is the federal government. Federal jobs—all acquired through Civil Service—are in the National Park Service, U.S. Forest Service and U.S. Fish and Wildlife Service. Salaries are listed in "GS" categories, the standard applied to all federal careers.

Beginning jobs tend to be the ones most directly associated with animals. Advancement in wildlife and conservation careers more often than not involves increasing amounts of laboratory and research work, and administration. It is strange indeed that advancement often means forsaking close contact with animals. At this point, where *up* means *out,* some workers in the animal field will go into a new area just to remain near animal life.

EDUCATION

For all but the most basic work, a bachelor's degree in wildlife biology, ecology or zoology is essential. Advancement in this field calls for advanced degrees, too. In high school you would concentrate on biology and the natural sciences. College will offer opportunities to specialize further—in wildlife and range management, ecology, forestry (because of its interaction with animals) and other areas. Research methodology is also extremely helpful, tieing in with the other study areas.

Seasonal employment and volunteering, discussed later in this chapter, provide on-site education as well as the opportunity to work in the field of your choice before you start college and during summer vacations.

Growing numbers of states require a bachelor's degree for work as forest or park rangers, fish and game control officers and assistant biologists. And since wildlife management and conservation deal with many state and federal regulations, an understanding of basic criminal justice and of animal laws and their enforcement is part of many jobs. This knowledge can be learned on the job as well as being part of your formal education.

For those of you who lack the time to attend classes in conservation or live too far away from schools offering such a curriculum, one answer may be a correspondence course.

The North American Correspondence Schools (with Administration Center in Pennsylvania and Curriculum Development offices in California) offer a Wildlife/Forestry conservation course to those attracted to outdoor careers. The course is approved by the California Superintendent of Public Education and the National Home Study Council.

The correspondence course offers study and guidance materials to prepare students for jobs in the conservation field. The School is quick to add that there are far more people seeking employment in this area than there are positions available. Robert D. Montgomery, the executive director, states that only 26.4% of the School's graduates find jobs, but he adds that the knowledge gained could work to the student's benefit further down the career-path. The testimonials of those who *did* find jobs after completing the course are impressive. One graduate stated that "the course gave me great confidence when I took the test for . . . conservation officer. Now I am next on the list to be hired."

The course includes study in game management, wildlife law enforcement, fish management and culture techniques, forest and park systems, forest protection, wildlife habitat and control and environmental protection. Lessons are assigned and graded, and students have up to two years to finish the course work. Consultation and career assistance services are available to graduates.

Sub-professional positions in conservation require a high school degree; senior positions generally require a college degree. In states where a bachelor's degree is mandated the correspondence course cannot substitute.

Although veterinary schools often concentrate on domestic animals, a fascinating exception is the Wildlife Service of the University of Pennsylvania's veterinary school. William Medway, the school's pathology professor, is the faculty advisor of this student-run clinic. Here, pigeons, gerbils, geese, finches and other injured or ill animals have been treated by the students. A five-year-old Bengal lizard named Big Red has been a patient. Anyone finding an injured wild bird or animal may bring it in 24 hours a day for treatment. There is no charge, but donations are appreciated. In a recent year, the clinic treated 160 wild creatures. This Wildlife Service is run by the first and second year veterinary students. Course credit is given. A term paper is required for full credit and encompasses such topics as how an owl tracks its prey. (Answer: through the auditory system.)

Do the captive, injured creatures take to their helpers? "They're not very appreciative of our efforts," said Jim Reed, one of the participating students. He feels the results are worth the effort, even though the creatures do not show affection or appreciation like domestic pets.

Legally-owned exotic animals are also treated at the clinic, for a fee. One visitor, a five-year-old parrot named Tillie, had plucked away her chest feathers from boredom. Her prescription? A change of diet, play toys—and repositioning Tillie's cage by a window and near a turned-on television! Other animals have been treated by every veterinary method from nail-clipping to antibiotics and major surgery.

WILDLIFE BIOLOGIST

The wildlife biologist is the one careerist who is most directly involved with the ongoing safety and well-being of wild animals. A wildlife biologist may spend days in winter camp, as Brad Allen, Randy Cross and others did northwest of Ashland, Maine during the winter of 1982. Allen and his teammates were on the trail of 50 hibernating black bears that they had fitted with radio-signaling collars the summer before. The biologists, working for the Maine Department of Inland Fisheries and Wildlife, tracked the bears to see how many had given birth to cubs, how many cubs they had apiece, and how healthy they appeared. They will use their data to estimate what the future black bear population will be.

In addition to learning about the habits and characteristics of black bears, their studies will help the state of Maine determine how many bears can—or should—legally be hunted without endangering the species. Since hunting is a multi-million-dollar business in the state, the team's research is important to the economy as well as to the animals.

In answer to an ever-louder "beep" signal, the team moved in on showshoes to a bear's hibernation spot, usually a ground-hollow or a brush-concealed hole. One team member covers the opening with a nylon net while another tranquilizes the bear with a gun on a pole. Then, they all carefully remove the bear— no easy job at 130 dead-weight pounds—and the cubs. These are kept warm in the biologists' jackets while they are weighed and their ears are tagged for later study. After weighing and recording, all the bears are replaced and the hole re-covered with underbrush to keep the cubs inside. The whole job has to be done in 45 minutes, the effective tranquilizer time.

The "bear study," as it is informally called, began in 1980 and will continue for some years until results are conclusive. Three teams of biologists work for three to four weeks in winter and for five months every spring and summer. Winter quarters are primitive, wood-heated cabins 25 miles from civilization in the Aroostook County woods. The only access to the outside world is by snowmobile.

Joanna Burger is a professor of biological sciences and director of the graduate ecology program at Rutgers University in New Brunswick, New Jersey. She also has a mission outside the classroom: preservation of the Least Tern, a tiny seashore bird on the state's endangered species list. Least Terns nest on beaches where their eggs are impossible to tell from pebbles—a protection against natural predators but not against people. Ms. Burger, working with a state tax grant, has protected nesting areas with snow fences and signs, and has tried to lure the birds to safer nesting spots with decoys. She has her work cut out for her; the birds are most vulnerable in July and August when the beaches are the most crowded. Since it is impossible to be everywhere at once, she has had to identify the ten largest nesting colonies along the Jersey Shore and limit her conservation efforts to them.

If you become a wildlife biologist, you may concentrate in one animal area as Brad Allen and Joanna Berger do, or you could work more generally in animal management. In any case, the biologist's work tends to be mission-oriented: basic observation and research aimed at solving or preventing problems related to wild animals and their habitats.

Habitat study is a key. One of the goals is to control the forest habitat to maintain the proper ecological balance of and for different creatures. If forest cutting is to be done, for instance, the wildlife biologist would work with foresters to decide what types of timber to be cut, where, and how much. Cutting large stands of mature timber would benefit species seeking new growth for cover or food, but at the expense of hawks, owls, woodpeckers and other creatures in need of older growth.

In a national forest where your work is coordinated with foresters and range managers, you may be the only wildlife biologist working with animals in a many-square-mile area of millions of acres. Census-taking, another frequent assignment, is often done by airplane, the best way to check changes in the population of ospreys, eagles and deer. In addition to coordinated efforts with foresters and others, a great deal of the wildlife biologist's work in national forests involves interrelationships with industry, lumbering and mining in permitted areas, to assure environmental protection.

The same basic tasks of animal management are performed by wildlife biologists in state forests, national parks and state parks. In parklands, however, the public is a factor and the interaction of animals and people—visitors, campers and hunters—is an important part of maintaining animal well-being through successful management of habitats and control of hunting volume.

Some biologists say half their time is spent in animal observation, banding and other direct involvement. The other half—and often a higher proportion of time—is taken up with recording, analyzing and reporting their findings and in related administrative detail.

One biologist whose time is largely taken up with travel is Dr. George Schaller of the New York Zoological Society. Dr. Schaller is a field worker—the ultimate wildlife biologist—and he is also a conservationist and zoologist. He has spent months, even years at a time, in such countries as Brazil, India, and Zaire. His job: researching wild animals and planning wildlife preserves for them.

Much of Dr. Schaller's work is funded by research grants from the National Geographic Society and similar organizations. A detailed field study—of snow leopards in the Himalayas, for instance—takes two to three years. Although Dr. Schaller usually works from a home base as close to the animals as possible and takes his family along to work with him, much time is spent in isolated field work. In Tanzania, his home base was 200 miles from the area he was observing, so a lot of tent camping was involved for him.

Dr. Schaller's work is more than pure research into animal habitats and conditions. Part of his goal is to work with local governments to design and establish preserves for protecting the wildlife he has studied. He has also written extensively and worked with wildlife-dedicated assistants in the host countries, teaching them how to conserve their own valuable wildlife.

Some 65% of wildlife biologists work for states, 20% for the federal government and the rest for universities, zoos, environmental groups and foundations. The relatively few available jobs usually go to those with advanced degrees. Beginners with bachelor's degrees earn from $9,000 to $11,000 a year; a senior biologist can earn up to $15,000.* Federally-employed biologists earn from $14,000 to $23,000; those with Ph.D. degrees earn more.

RANGERS

Rangers are employed by national and state parks. Their duties are similar in both facilities, and there is some overlap with tasks performed by wildlife biologists and wildlife conservation officers.

---

*From *Careers Working with Animals: the Humane Society's Guide* by Guy R. Hodge.

Park rangers and their supervisors have the most direct control over park lands, the animals who live there and the visitors who come there. The ranger welcomes visitors, assigns campsites, collects fees, reports on weather, conducts nature walks and campfire lectures—and answers every question from "Will the bears bother me?" to "Where can I get ice?"

The ranger is also a police officer of sorts whose duties include making the public aware of park rules and seeing to it they are obeyed. Where hunting and fishing are permitted, this job is more often done by the wildlife conservation officer.

Another element of ranger life is overseeing the general condition of the park. Are fences mended? Trails neat and well-marked? Parking areas clean? Campsites ready for occupancy? Rangers patrol all areas of the park, noting what work must be done and assigning it to conservation crews, often young seasonal workers or volunteers. Ranger duties may take you far away from the public and may involve long periods out-of-doors, patrolling by 4WD vehicle or on horseback.

Along with the people- and park-care elements of the job, rangers are front-line animal care workers, too. A ranger must have an intimate knowledge of the park's wildlife mixture and the visitors' impact on it, of weather conditions and their potential effects on the animals, and of what steps to take toward successful animal management. Along with the wildlife biologist, the ranger surveys wildlife and reports on its conditions, provides animals with water and food in times of severe weather, rescues animals found in difficulties, and traps animals to move them to distant locations where food supplies are better or where visitors will not go.

The answer to "Will the bears bother me?" might just be "Yes" if conditions are wrong. When bears and other predators cannot find food in the wild, they may raid campsites—not a good state of affairs. By taking positive action in advance, the rangers and their assistants can maintain the proper balance in the park between people and the natural environment.

The forest ranger and range manager are related careers, but less related to people and animals. Forest rangers monitor environmental and man-made conditions in national and state forests. While these duties include a degree of animal care, it is secondary to the over-all preservation of forest lands, the control or direction of logging where it is permitted, and general management of thousands of acres of uninhabited wilderness.

Range managers perform much the same duties, but in addition they interact with ranchers who may be permitted to use the open rangelands for grazing cattle. The range manager helps determine the amount of grazing that may be done, and works with ranchers to maintain the size of the herd and the size and location of available acreage.

Starting salaries for these careers are about $10,000 to $12,000 for degreed applicants and can be as high as $15,000. Additional degrees mean added earnings; a range manager, for example, with a year or more of graduate study can earn $18,500. Salaries will vary by state.

WILDLIFE CONSERVATION OFFICER

Titles such as *wildlife conservation officer, conservation warden* or—most usually in the public mind—*game warden* all describe the same state government position. In federal government work for the U.S. Fish and Wildlife Service the title is *special agent.*

Originally the job was one purely of enforcement of hunting and fishing laws. Today the job still involves the regulation of game animals (mammals, birds, and fishes) including investigation and enforcement, and there is also increasing overlap with the tasks of other conservation workers.

Today, as a wildlife conservation officer, you would check licenses, regulate catches and enforce applicable laws—but you may also help conduct animal surveys, do rescue work, operate feeding stations, relocate animals and may even be involved in fire detection and monitoring state and private game breeding farms. Like the park ranger, you may also speak before civic-minded hunting and fishing groups, providing safety information and emphasizing the need for conservation to their audiences.

Federal special agents are primarily enforcement officers, performing a broad range of regulatory duties from granting federal wildlife permits to flying enforcement patrols.

As with growing numbers of conservation workers, education past high school is becoming more important as a requirement for the limited number of available jobs. And several states have physical requirements that must be met. Experience in some phases of wildlife management and conservation or law enforcement is decidedly helpful. Federal special agents must have a bachelor's degree in wildlife biology or criminal justice, or at least its equivalent in job-related experience.

State starting salaries range from $7,000 to above $10,000; GS-5 is the usual starting grade in the federal system for special agents, but those with unusual experience may begin at GS-7 or GS-9. Advancement to GS-14 is possible. State-employed officers may advance similarly but advancement is difficult since jobs are hard to come by. As this game-oriented activity expands to include non-game (wildlife) work, the field may expand slightly.

SEASONAL WORK AND VOLUNTEERING

This is the best way to get your feet wet—literally—in the field of wildlife management and conservation work. Seasonal workers, usually given living quarters and board, plus a small salary, are employed by many states, and there are several federally-funded, paid, and volunteer programs that use young people for outdoor work in parks and forests.

The work, as you might expect, is largely physical. Seasonal workers and volunteers may perform the day-to-day maintenance and repair jobs in parks and forests—everything from digging firebreaks to marking trails. Also, they may assist rangers and other full-time workers in animal management, enforcement, census-taking...in any job that has to be done. The very variety of the work is its virtue. A summer or two between high school and college, or earlier (the Youth Conservation Corps accepts summer workers as young as age 15) will let you know whether or not a career in wildlife management is for you.

These summer jobs will also give you the learn-by-doing experience that most government agencies consider as valuable as formal education.

In addition to paid seasonal park and forest programs offered by many states, national programs include:

- *Youth Conservation Corps* (YCC)—40,000 members; 1,000 projects; ages 15-18; 4 to 10 weeks (average, 8); average $13/day salary. YCC, Box 2975, Washington DC 20013.

- *Job Corps Civilian Conservation Center*—largely vocational job training, some conservation work. JCCC c/o your State Employment Service or Director, Manpower Training and Youth Activities, OMB, USDI, Washington DC 20242.

- *National Park Service*—very limited seasonal work; preference given to previous seasonal workers and veterans. Pamphlet, "Seasonal Employment," from

Personnel Office, National Park Service, USDI, Washington DC 20240.

- *Forest Service*—limited employment; must be 18 for most openings. Applications available from most Forest Service offices.

- *Youth Conservation Corps*—8,000 summer camp staff jobs; minimum age 19; natural science background; previous experience working with youth. Same address as JCCC above.

- *Young Adult Conservation Corps*—similar to YCC; ages 16-23; preference given to people in high unemployment areas; 22,000 jobs offered. YACC c/o your State Employment Service or same address as JCCC above.

- *Federal Fish and Wildlife positions*—part- and full-time. Apply to Civil Service Commission, 1900 E Street NW, Washington DC 20415.

The logical alternative if paid jobs are not available is volunteering. Among the volunteer opportunities for summer work are:

- *Student Conservation Association*—Box 550, Charlestown NH 03603.

- *Volunteers in Parks*—age 18, younger with parental consent. Use standard form 170 to apply, available from any Post Office. Pamphlet, "Volunteering in Parks," USDI, Washington DC 20242.

- *Volunteers in Forests*—same age requirements as above. Pamphlet, "Forest Service Volunteer" with application available from U.S. Forest Service, USDA, Washington DC 20250.

CAREERS IN CONSERVATION

The conservation movement is largely the province of a variety of private foundations and organizations. While some are conservation-minded in a general way, many are single-issue organizations dedicated to preserving such creatures as seals or whales, or to maintaining marshlands or wilderness areas against the onslaught of commercial animal exploitation or industrial takeover.

Although their financing is a relative drop in the bucket compared to government spending for forests, parks and wildlife and conservation, the 14 "club member" environmental organizations with Washington lobbies wield a surprising amount of influence and throw an increasing number of dollars into the environmental fight. This group, called the "green lobby" by *Fortune* magazine, boasts a combined membership of 5,415,000 Americans—one person in 42 is a contributor—and fielded a combined 1982 budget of $92.9 million, with the giant National Wildlife Federation alone accounting for 4,200,000 members and $37.1 million in funds.

Not all groups are animal-related; their concerns range from furthering solar energy to fighting corporate pollution. And the "club" does not include the many smaller single-issue organizations, zoological societies, humane organizations and local SPCAs.

All of these advocacy groups offer opportunities for caring people although direct contact with animals is limited at best. Only super-activist organizations like Greenpeace send people into nature to go literally head-to-head against animal slaughterers. But they do offer career opportunities for people willing to work for their causes indirectly.

Among these specialists are professional lobbyists whose role is to influence legislators favorably toward their causes, local, regional and national. Other advocates approach the task through the legal process, studying environmental and animal regulations and working with legislators to create more favorable legislation, to strengthen the laws that exist, and to work against their pro-industry lobbying counterparts.

A major role is fund-raising among individuals and environmentally-concerned corporations. People who would ordinarily be involved in the sales and marketing of consumer products and services instead devote their abilities to "selling" the "product" of the environmental group for whom they work, marketing their group's philosophy just as they would any other commodity—with equal skill and dedication.

Within each organization just as in any industrial company are the "troops"—those who create the communications, open the mail, answer the telephones, keep the books, run the computers and do every other kind of office job—but for a cause they believe to be more important than marketing automobiles or promoting motion pictures.

Not all work, however, is office-based or centered in Washington, DC. The Nature Conservancy, for instance, although headquartered across the Potomac in Arlington, Virginia, is a mushrooming organization that now owns some 700 private nature preserves nationwide. But land ownership and management is not its primary goal. TNC has been extremely successful in buying open land and reselling it to dedicated corporations which are as intent in its preservation as the Conservancy. TNC also markets land to local environmental groups which repay its cost through private fund-raising. It has acquired land which it has turned over to many states under similar preservation arrangements. So far, the 145,000-member organization has saved some two million acres.

TNC deeply feels its responsibilities in managing the land it owns. It employs a corps of environmental and wildlife biologists, range and land managers and enforcement people. Their training and work are very similar to the jobs performed in state and national preserves: maintaining the balance of nature; preserving endangered species; controlling hunting, fishing and camping in lands where these activities are permitted. TNC employs corporate and individual fund-raisers, land acquisition specialists and others whose business is preserving the past to protect the future.

For information about TNC, write to their headquarters at 1800 North Kent Street, Arlington VA 22209.

TNC also welcomes volunteers, as does any nonprofit corporation or environmental group. Volunteering your time and talent may well be a way to acquire experience that will eventually pay off in preservation- or animal-related employment.

Volunteering can be equally rewarding for the professional who can give of time and ability. Marlin Perkins is one such passionate animal protectionist. The Director Emeritus of the St. Louis Zoo and co-producer of the acclaimed TV series, *Wild Kingdom,* Perkins is a highly vocal and effective advocate of animal protection. He defends the modern zoo, citing numerous examples of the zoo's role in preventing the extinction of many species, and criticizes shortsighted policies such as the wholesale slaughter of wolves. With the wolves largely gone, problems such as overabundance of elk in places like Yellowstone National Park have been the result. So strongly does Marlin Perkins feel on this subject that he and his wife, Carol, are working to create a natural sanctuary for wolves just a few miles from their St. Louis home.

Dr. Harold Albers, a Florida veterinarian and past President of the Pinellas County Veterinary Medical Association, has become an expert on the treatment of oil-damaged waterfowl, and contributes his time and knowledge at many conferences on this and other aspects of animal management. He has involved oil companies in the problem with excellent results, and has developed a bird rehabilitation manual now widely used by groups such as Florida's Associated Marine Institutes and

International Bird Rescue. With 9,000 miles of coastland in need of preservation and protection with limited funds, the state of Florida needs the help of dedicated people like Dr. Albers.

COMMUNICATIONS

There are varied opportunities in communications for the animal care worker, although these are often combined with other duties.

In both national and state parks, the park rangers develop and conduct tours, lectures, and nature walks which usually emphasize wildlife and conservation. They may also create and produce park information leaflets, brochures and tourist information to distribute to park visitors.

In zoos and safari parks, especially those catering to children (of all ages), assistant curators or skilled animal keepers may prepare live animal exhibits and also run a children's zoo. Nearly every zoo also has a public relations person who writes brochures and prepares talks on the animals. These same people, or other staffers, may be animal photographers who prepare the pictures for slide shows, publicity releases, and brochures.

Conservation organizations also use the services of skilled communications people who prepare fund-raising and consciousness-raising materials for direct mail solicitation and awareness programs. Some organizations have staff people to prepare communications while others either share this responsibility with outside advertising and public relations firms, or turn all such work over to them.

Although they are relatively rare, there are full-time journalists and photographers whose careers are largely or entirely concerned with animals.

Competition is keen for just about all communications assignments. Since the communications person may have to wear other organizational hats as well, your possibilities of working in animal communications are improved if you have excellent writing and verbal skills, knowledge of layout and design, plus photographic or illustrative capabilities as well as a thorough knowledge of the animals with which you work—plus a well-developed ability to talk on your feet and make a good impression on the public.

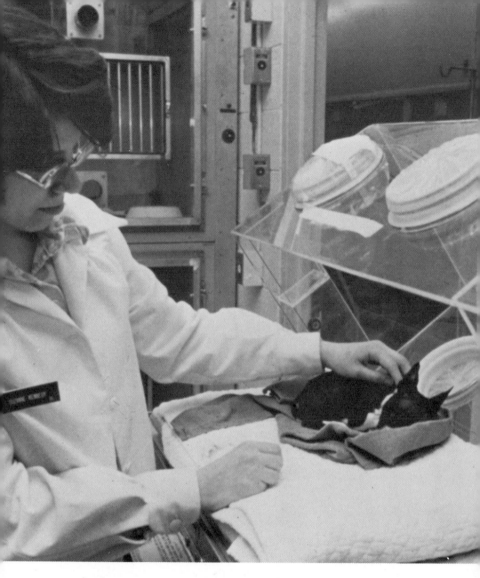

Incubators are used in veterinary practice much as they are in human medical practice. Photo: Michigan State University, College of Veterinary Medicine, Animal Technology Program and North American Veterinary Technician Association.

CHAPTER 13

CAREERS WITH DOGS: FROM OUTSIDE JOB TO SELF-EMPLOYMENT

Man's best friend offers many opportunities for young people to carve interesting careers. Almost everyone starting in the field works for someone else, but experience, initiative, a developing business sense and an ability to get along well with people can result in a successful career working for yourself. Many is the dog groomer, kennel assistant, or veterinary hospital aide who has gone on to establish her or his own boarding kennel, obedience school or professional handling clientele.

COMBINATION CAREERS

The primary dog-related careers are kennel owner, breeder, groomer, trainer, and handler. Many people combine two or more areas of expertise in a single career. A kennel owner may board and groom dogs for customers, and may also breed dogs for sale or conduct obedience classes for dogs and their owners.

As we discuss the careers individually, keep in mind the possibilities of combining one or more—one alone may not provide enough income.

Remember, too, that all dog-related careers call for a high degree of "that special something" we've mentioned earlier: the innate, almost instinctive ability to relate strongly to animals, to understand them and in turn to be understood (and not be fooled!) by them. Dogs, like other creatures, know almost instantly, as little children do, who is on their wavelength and who is not. Professional "dog people" are almost universal in their belief that this trait is a gift rather than something that can be learned; either you have it or you don't. Even limited experience with dogs will point the way for you in this respect.

EDUCATIONAL AND PHYSICAL REQUIREMENTS

Much dog-related activity is learned by doing, although there are a few schools that offer training in such areas as dog grooming and kennel management. The best way to learn is to start as an apprentice or helper to someone in one of the career areas. High school courses in biology and the natural sciences are a help, as is a basic understanding of animal health. Happy experience with your own dog is a good beginning, too.

There are some physical demands. Lots of work is involved. Large dogs can be hefty and cumbersome—and they won't climb onto their own three-foot-high grooming tables!

KENNEL WORK—THE ENTREE

Working in a breeding or boarding kennel is probably the best entree to any career with dogs. As a kennel worker, you may be short on money, but you can expect to be long on experience—kennel work is the closest thing to total canine immersion.

The things you do will be varied. You may be called upon to prepare dry dog food or cut up meat for meals, keep cages and runs clean and fresh, fill water bowls, exercise the dogs, help with nail-clipping, brushing, washing and grooming chores, and answer the telephone. If yours is a boarding kennel, you may also sign in visiting pets, record and collect their boarding fees, note their food preferences, where their owners can be reached in case of emergency, and check the pets out when they are departing.

If you work for a breeding kennel you can expect, in addition to all the customary kennel chores, to assist with breeding and birthing, and perhaps to show puppies to prospective buyers. If yours is a kennel that teaches obedience courses or is involved in the dog show circuit, you may help with the training classes or go along on the busy weekend show tours—a job that means hours of driving or flying, taking care of the pets en route, helping with their grooming on arrival at the show, and packing everything up again for the trip home, or to the next show— some exhibitors attend two shows in one weekend.

You could be doing all of the above—indeed, total immersion!

In the process, there's a lot to know, and you would be learning it the best possible way: under the watchful eyes of those who know the subject intimately, and who would have something new to teach you almost every hour of the day. You would learn the finer points of removing burrs from a dog's shaggy coat, and perhaps the ins-and-outs of dog obedience training. You may learn what the proper conformation (physical characteristics and appearance) should be for one or more breeds, and what show judges look for, in ring judging and obedience trials, from the dog and its handler. You'd learn the basics of dog feeding and care, and at least some of the rudiments of veterinary medicine and the recognition of dog health problems. You would soon catch on to what kennel temperatures are right for different breeds—room temperature for most small dogs, less for outdoor breeds—and the right way to get a dog to swallow a pill.

Most important, you would learn whether or not operating a kennel is your idea of a lifetime career, or if more specialized work with dogs is best for you.

Harris Dunlap's Zero Kennels

Harris Dunlap of Bakers Mills, New York, is a kennel operator whose hobby—racing sled dogs—became the basis for his career. His Zero Kennels, which he operates as a family business, is the largest associated with this unique sport.

Dunlap's interest began shortly after he finished his college training as an artist. He bought a Siberian Husky as a pet, and added a war surplus dogsled. His activity has grown with the sport, which has boomed in the last 20 years. Now, Harris Dunlap wins prize money—from $15,000 to $20,000 a year—in dogsled races, and earns considerably more by breeding, training, and selling his own breed of sled dogs. A top-performing team lead dog is worth as much as $5,000.

Racing sled dogs is a rugged life, especially in the 100-day racing season that starts every New Year's Day. Dunlap and his teams may travel 20,000 miles in this time to compete in races as long as 1,171 miles that are held in winter settings as far away as Alaska. His usual entourage is 36 racing dogs plus sleds, equipment and crew.

Dunlap's own dogs, which he spends the rest of the year breeding and training, are specially bred by him for racing. The breed is based on the Siberian Husky, but other traits have been bred in, vascular strength and stamina, for instance. Stamina is the essential element of the sled dog: each dog runs about 1,500 miles in training and competition during the racing season. Of his 36 racing dogs, 20 are lead dogs, extra-intelligent animals capable of interpreting the driver's wishes to the team dogs by a combination of instinct and example. Because the mental and physical pressures are considerable, the lead dogs are rotated frequently, but never during a race. Race rules have it that dogs may be removed from a team but new ones cannot be substituted.

Dunlap's talent for breeding and racing sled dogs paid off in 1983 when his team won the World Sled Dog Championship, to cap a string of first and second place finishes for the season.

The Kennel Business

As a beginning kennel worker, you would need no financial investment for a salaried job. As you gain experience, a bit of paid time off, occasional bonuses for extra hours worked, and even a profit-sharing arrangement may come your way.

A salaried, experienced kennel worker employed full-time and with living accommodations provided may earn $12,000 or more a year. The accommodations should be considered "plus" income when they are included.

If you decide to operate your own kennel, you will have to scout for a suitable location to buy or rent in an area where kennels are acceptable, and decide which canine services you should offer. What you earn will be governed by your overhead, versus your charges for the services you give, and the volume your kennel attracts. A good business sense and an outgoing personality, important to the kennel worker, are essential ingredients for success in your own kennel business.

DOG GROOMER

Debbie Weiss, owner and sole operator of Debbie's Dog Grooming Salon in Elkins Park, Pennsylvania, finds her work very creative. "A dog may come in in a total mess," she says. "I groom him and make him feel better." This is her motivation—her work makes *her* feel good, too.

Creating what she calls "creature comfort" is not easy. A total grooming involves careful combing-out of the coat—often with considerable thinning and clipping—as the first step. Nails may be clipped, too, something many dogs fail to appreciate while it's going on. Nor do they relish ear-cleaning. Then it's into the bath, and the reaction to this depends on the dog. Some love it, others express different opinions! After a thorough, careful drying, often done with drying equipment that dries the fur but does not dry-out the skin or allow the dog to become chilled, comes further brushing, thinning, clipping and styling. The final touch may be a bit of scent, and the job is done.

A dog groomer may operate an independent business as Debbie does, or work for a kennel owner or in a grooming salon. Since it's strictly "piece work," volume is the key to making it work financially. Since overhead—rent, heat, light and advertising—are fixed expenses, the grooming operation not associated with a kennel has to be brisk to be successful. A groomer who works for a kennel may be in a fairly good position since there are always other things to do if the grooming part of the business is slow.

The groomer who works for an established shop usually does so on commission, much as a beautician does. This is normally 50% of what the shop charges the customer; thus, earnings will vary with the shop's volume. $30 to $40 a day is the average earning rate for groomers—more when they become proficient and if the shop is a busy one.

Opening a grooming shop means that you as owner can earn more than you could as an employee. But doing so also means making an investment of as much as $4,000 for signs, reception area, grooming tables and tools, cages, driers, rent deposit and utility connection charges—plus, of course, the continuing overhead expenses. Shop owners say that among the elements needed for success are an accessible location in a busy neighborhood with easy parking and a consistent advertising program. A good listing in the Yellow Pages is mentioned by many. If you have established a good reputation as a groomer with another nearby kennel or salon, you may have some built-in following when you open your doors. Your chances would be even better if you were lucky enough to be able to buy out or buy into a going shop, perhaps the one for which you work.

One of the few schools for dog grooming in the country is in Philadelphia, Pennsylvania. The Pennsylvania School of Dog Grooming is licensed by the state and offers basic, advanced and professional courses for "...that special someone with a lot of patience and a great love and compassion for animals." Another school, this one in California, offers a 15-week course with a total of 600 classroom hours. Live—often lively—subjects, including an occasional cat, are used to teach every element of the craft.

TRAINING CAREERS

In addition to their value as pets, many dogs are bred and trained for work. Others are trained just to be nicer to have around—no unscheduled barking, jumping into laps, or bedroom-slipper breakfasts. And many dogs are carefully trained for performance in the show ring and the obedience trial field. While some canine skills are instinctive—Sheepdogs, for instance, seem to be born knowing what to do with sheep—most must be taught by people.

Different training goals call for specific knowledge, but all dog trainers have many traits in common. Their patience, for one thing, must be almost infinite. Dogs are highly intelligent and retain knowledge well once it is given to them, but the giving calls for extreme patience plus consistency and kindness. Firmness, too, is part of the trainer's makeup, but firmness always applied in a gentle and consistent way. Dogs thrive on appreciation; even when a dog does something wrong and is made to understand this, the impression from the trainer must be a kindly one.

The Leader Dog Trainers

Most all trainers, whether schooling dogs in obedience, training them to lead the blind, or to be part of a law enforcement team, must be people-oriented as well as animal-oriented. This is certainly true of the 20 full-time trainers (among a staff of 56) who work at the headquarters of Leader Dogs for the Blind® of Rochester, Michigan.

Leader Dogs for the Blind is funded primarily by the Lions International, a service organization dedicated to aiding the blind. Even the dogs are contributed. They are usually German Shepherds, Laborador and Golden Retrievers, and are always female, because they have proved to be more temperamentally suited to the work than males.

When the dogs arrive at Rochester, they are trained for five months by the trainers. As part of their own training, the trainers are often blindfolded, to appreciate firsthand what it is like to be dependent on a dog for guidance.

A dog to be trained as a Leader Dog will first learn to wear the shoulder harness that is its contact with the blind person. The dog must learn that she's "on duty" whenever this harness is in place. One by one, with constant constant repetition, the instructor repeats the commands that the blind person will use, and teaches the dog the correct response to each one. The dog is taught to stop, to go forward, and to go right or left on command. Most important, it is taught to stop at every curb, even the wheelchair curbs that are flush with the street. In time, the dogs learn not to go forward into traffic—but the blind owner must take the responsibility for the dog's reactions to commands; that is, the owner must listen for vehicles and learn to sense the flow of people around her or him in city traffic and thus know when streets can be crossed. This work takes time and infinite patience—small wonder that training the guide dog takes several months before it meets its new owner.

Thirty-two human candidates at a time live at the Leader Dog facility, and work closely and harmoniously with their dogs and trainers. After a get-acquainted period the match of dog and candidate is evaluated by the trainer.

The "schooling" of the new owner takes four weeks. First, the dog learns that total allegiance goes not to the trainer that she knows but to the new master that she does not. The dog learns, too, that she can relax and simply be a pet and companion when the shoulder harness is replaced with a leash. Work time is over, and the command words for duty are never used when the dog is out of harness. Dog and master live as one during the training.

Every day, in good weather and bad—Leader Dog applicants are forewarned about winter Michigan weather!—dog, master and trainer practice the commands and movements over and over. A major lesson is learning to respond to the master's commands. As confidence grows, candidates, trailed discreetly by the trainers, move from the grounds of the Leader Dog facility into the small-town traffic of Rochester. Traffic situations are slowly added as familiarity and confidence are established—and before "graduation," the rush of nearby Detroit traffic is taken in stride. The trainers teach city-bound dogs and owners to cope with such special conditions as elevators, revolving doors, train and bus steps, and subway stations.

Dogs are taught never to cross streets diagonally but only from one curb to the opposing one—a degree of consistency that is essential to the blind person's confidence in maintaining proper orientation in city traffic.

In an article, "Free to Travel," Leader Dog® training is explained this way: "The orientation and mobility program...deals with the areas of body image, gait, coordination, position and awareness of location. The...program attempts to look at each person as an individual, assess the handicap, and plan a program to insure effective and efficient travel."

It is the trainer's responsibility to train the candidate just as completely as he or she trains the dog so the two become a team. More than 300 teams are trained each year; more than 6,400 have graduated since the school's founding in 1939.

Once on their own, the dog is "guided" by the blind person to the extent that he or she knows how many streets to cross, and in which direction, to get from point A to point B, and to return. In time and with practice, dog and owner can follow the same course to and from work or from home to the neighborhood store, with a pleasantly relaxed interdependence. In one sense, the training never ends.

Another never-ending consideration is the relationship of dog and master. Leader Dogs for the Blind and similar organizations teach the new masters the same degree of kindness and consistency to which the dogs respond during training—and they usually follow-up afterward to see how the relationship is progressing. Most of the dog and master teams adjust well—a tribute to the quality of the trainers' work and the dedication of all concerned.

Any blind person over age 16 with the ability and temperament to care for a dog is eligible for a Leader Dog. There is no charge; the average cost of $6,000 for each dog and its training is paid for by donations, primarily from Lions Club chapters.

Although it is the largest organization of its kind, Leader Dogs for the Blind is one of several devoted to training dogs for blind people. The Seeing Eye and International Guiding Eyes are two others.

Jobs as trainers of dogs for the blind are neither plentiful nor well-paying. Apprenticeship to a recognized organization is the usual method of entering this specialized training field. Most apprentices should have had at least a year of previous work experience in another area of dog management, as a veterinary assistant, kennel worker or obedience trainer. Since the job calls for instilling confidence in the dogs and their masters, you as a trainer must have confidence in yourself, and be as dedicated to people as you are to animals. Apprenticeship may last as long as three years. Earnings vary from $650 to $1,100 a month; full-time work after apprenticeship pays somewhat more.

One way in which you could contribute to this cause is to raise a donor pup through the 4-H Club program (see Chapter 4). After a year or more of home life, the 4-H dogs are given to The Seeing Eye in Morristown, NJ.

The K-9 Dog Trainer

German Shepherds, diligent, responsive and intelligent in their work with the blind, exhibit these tendencies—plus a few others—in police work. The K-9 trainer, like the guide dog trainer, works with young, grown dogs, teaching them to wade head-first into trouble—but only on command! The police dog trainer works at the same time to train the police officer who will be the dog's teammate throughout its law enforcement career. This takes place only after the dog has been thoroughly screened to make sure it is not gun-shy—or worse—crowd-shy.

It took 14 weeks of training before Abington Township (Pennsylvania) police officers Douglas Mealo and Robert Mann and their dogs, Zak and Duke, graduated from the nearby Philadelphia Police Academy with K-9 credentials. Both officers quickly proved the value of their dogs. Officer

Mealo and Zak headed off what their commanding officer characterized as "a potential riot" just by appearing before an unruly mob. Officer Mann did even better on a similar occasion: the sound of Duke's barking and the sight of the police van rocking were enough to convince a crowd that it suddenly had better places to be. In investigating a reported home robbery, Zak found—and held—two suspects under a bed until Officer Mealo could arrest them.

As is the custom with K-9 dogs, Zak and Duke live with their officers. The two suburban Philadelphia Policemen agree with other K-9 officers that their love of animals was the reason why they volunteered for K-9 duty.

The 14-week K-9 course given by the Philadelphia Police Academy for its own officers and those of nearby towns is typical. Officer and dog learn together. A command such as "Watch' em" or "Bark" is the dog's cue to act aggressively—to snarl, bark, bare its teeth and strain at its leash. Unless commanded to be aggressive, K-9 dogs are alert but quiet and well-mannered. By contrast, they will actually attack when commanded to do so if the officer thinks the situation calls for it.

As with dogs for the blind, the early part of the training is taken up with building mutual confidence between officer and dog—and making sure before the training gets too far that the chemistry is right between them—a job that calls for acute observation and experience on the trainer's part. Then, as with the blind, command and response are replayed until commands are obeyed instantly, consistently and dependably.

After the teams start police duty, the dogs are kept sharp by continued training in procedures taught by the Academy trainers. There may be a period each day or two when officers and their dogs practice attack procedures, with other officers playing the parts of criminal suspects. Since the dogs are taught never to attack someone in uniform, padded jackets are the "uniforms" worn by the "criminals" during these exercises.

Despite the cost of the dogs and their training and the time away from active duty needed to train a K-9 team, more police departments are realizing the benefits of K-9 patrols. A K-9 team can control even a large crowd far more effectively than several officers—and with far less chance of trouble. And most K-9 dogs can sniff out hidden drugs or people, jobs the officers cannot do as well, or at all.

K-9 dog trainers are schooled in basic obedience training, plus the specifics of their profession. Some K-9 dogs are trained on contract by people who raise and train security dogs. And the opportunity to become a K-9 police officer is another potential career with dogs.

Security Dog Trainers

Security dogs are a related specialty, but their training is not as comprehensive as K-9 training. These, too, are usually the breeds that most people are a bit wary of encountering, German Shepherds and Dobermans. They are generally not trained to attack, but are schooled to bark and snarl ferociously when approached by someone other than their owner on the property they are guarding. Some are trained to attack.

Security dogs are sometimes rented by the companies that use them. The kennel owner-trainer who specializes in security dogs has a long day. It starts with picking up the dogs in the morning when the factories, lumberyards, or stores where the dogs patrol are about to open, returning them to their kennels, feeding and caring for them. Through the day when the work dogs sleep, the trainer may work with new dogs or teach obedience classes. As evening approaches, the guard dogs go back to their respective locations for another night of duty.

Although the dogs don't patrol, they don't snooze on the job, either. Their hearing is so acute that they can swiftly and noisily respond to any sound.

The kennel operator who gives rented security dogs their basic training may also be a supplier of trainable or partially-trained dogs to police departments. This business person may also sell security dogs—again, usually the breeds that people tend to distrust—to people who feel they need the protection of such dogs at home or on a lonely city job. Or such a person can train client's dogs in security techniques or general obedience.

A dog obedience trainer may also hold classes for dogs and their owners without involving themselves in the overhead and responsibilities of kennel operation. Some trainers are able to operate with little business overhead beyond advertising expense and the cost of renting a hall or gym, or an open field. Others operate kennels, or work for kennel owners.

Investment and Income

With so many areas of dog training to consider, it should come as no surprise that the trainer's investment (in time if not in dollars) and earnings vary widely. Hourly rates of $10 and more for individual obedience training, or $10 to $25 for each group class of 1 to 1½ hours' length are usual. As a full-time trainer, you can expect yearly earnings ranging from $6,000 to $25,000 or more, depending on your reputation, size of classes and types of training. For instance, if your skills include advanced obedience in American Kennel Club categories, you will command excellent earnings if your canine clients are able to climb the ladder of AKC proficiency. The steps are: Companion Dog; Companion Dog Excellent; Utility Dog and Utility Dog Tracking. Each is more complex than the last, and the trainer able to excel in this rarified atmosphere is rewarded accordingly.

DOG BREEDER

The American Kennel Club (AKC) recognizes 128 distinct dog breeds. Not everyone who buys a purebred dog is interested in showing it—the vast majority just want a good pet with certain characteristics—but the whole dog show scene is big business. From the prestigious Westminster which could be called the Show of Shows on down to local events, AKC-sanctioned dog shows attract thousands of exhibitors and their would-be champion dogs. The action is non-stop; a breeder could attend one or two shows every weekend of the year.

The dog breeder whose stock earns the blue ribbons and silver trophies naturally commands far more money for puppies than the one who does not win in competition or who chooses not to compete at all. The element of gain, plus a hefty dose of ego-satisfaction, are at the root of most championship quests.

The keys to breeding success are a knowledge of breed bloodlines and conformation, and the ability to produce puppies in a healthy environment. Acquiring breeding knowledge takes time and experience, usually with one breed, sometimes with two or more. For each mating, the bloodlines and ancestry of past generations on both sides must be studied with care. All past champions are considered in light of the laws of heredity. Since these laws are not absolute, judgment enters the picture: "How good a litter would we get if we bred Champion Lilli von Austerlitz of Grendview with our Champion Ludwig von Wienerschnitzel?" The hope, of course, would be a litter of pups at least some of which would exhibit the finest characteristics of both parents, and all of which would be eminently marketable to Dachshund fanciers.

As a dog breeder who tackles the show circuit, you must be prepared to spend considerable amounts of time and money to compete. The show drill involves infinitely careful feeding and grooming of the dogs to be shown—grooming that begins well before the exhibition and continues up to the second before the handler (who may or may not be the breeder-owner) parades the dog for its magic moment before the judges. The dogs must be carefully caged for transport, fed, tended and kept at their peak en route. And detailed training in show etiquette must take place before a dog is exhibited for the first time.

There's an interesting analogy between dog shows and vintage automobile exhibitions, a subject the authors know firsthand. Just as a Classic Car must be shown in as close to its original, as-new condition as possible with points deducted from a theoretical 100 score for flaws spotted by the judges, a show dog must appear to be as close to the ideal example of its breed as possible. And, just as a car owner-exhibitor may feel a certain judge doesn't know Auburn 851 upholstery pleats as well as he or she should, dog exhibitors, too, may complain about judging results. The AKC is working to establish written qualification tests for judges; these have not existed until now. To make the analogy complete, there are no written tests for vintage car judges, either.

But, complaints aside, judges are licensed by AKC and they know the breeds they are asked to judge. While some may have quirks of subjective judgment that add a factor of luck to judging, the vast majority are qualified and fair.

Even though a dog breeder may choose not to show, a professional works to maintain quality through careful selection— always with AKC-registered stock—to assure continuity of the breed and satisfaction for buyers.

Dog breeding can be a home industry for the family that mates its AKC-registered female with a similarly registered male and then sells its purebred puppies for anything from $150 to $500 each on up to the climate-controlled, Championship-showing, nationally advertised kennel that turns out future champions on a large scale for large dollars. But home- or kennel-based breeders all customarily provide the AKC

registration for their puppies, and raise them in healthy surroundings. Puppies should be kept until well past weaning time
and should be wormed, inoculated and OK'd by a veterinarian
before being offered for sale.

A dog breeder who operates a kennel, or a kennel operator of
any kind, must comply with local zoning. Dogs may have to be
kept indoors after certain hours, and noise may have to be
controlled. For this reason, many kennel owners are in the
country or suburbs, and those that primarily sell puppies find
this is not a deterrent to business. Nearness to a community is,
however, a prerequisite for a kennel that is run primarily for
boarding and grooming.

SHOW DOG HANDLER

This is a glamor career with dogs—but behind the glitter lies
the grit: long hours, much travel, lengthy apprenticeship and
detailed knowledge.

Any AKC member in good standing can, of course, show his
or her own dog in the ring or in obedience trials. But just as the
owners of a racehorse hire a jockey to ride for the winner's
circle because he's the best, so owners of championship dogs
turn over their leashes to professional handlers who often have
what it takes to bring out the best there is in a dog.

The leading 300 or so handlers are members of the Professional Handler's Association, a select organization with its own
standards of ethics and performance. Members must have had
at least five years' professional handling experience, must pub-
lish handling fees for their clients, and must have high personal
and financial standing.

A skilled handler can earn up to $75,000 a year or more—but
he or she works hard for it. A handler can travel to 100 or more
shows a year, ranging from Canada to South America and

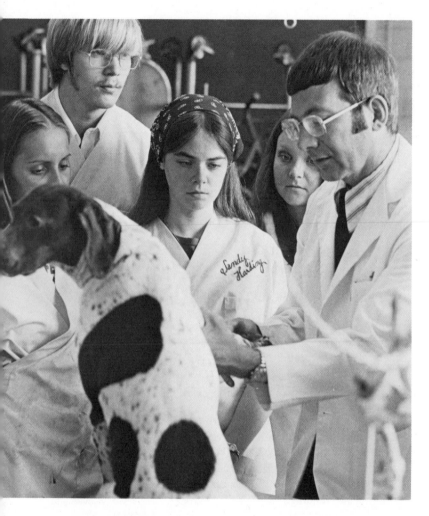

Much small-animal veterinary practice involves a knowledge of dogs and their particular needs. Photo: Courtesy of Purdue University Medical Illustration, School of Veterinary Medicine; Sam Roger, photographer.

anywhere in the United States. The handler who takes clients' dogs on each trip is entirely responsible for their care and grooming beforehand, en route, during the show and on the return.

In addition to having the "certain something" that commands both love and respect from dogs, you as a handler must have "done time"—years of it—in dog obedience, grooming, nutrition and health care. Many handlers also operate kennels, often with obedience schools as part of the operation.

A few handlers are obedience specialists, working with dogs that may not have the conformation to do well in the show ring, but animals that have the "heart" and intelligence to score high in obedience trials. Most handlers specialize in show judging, working skillfully and smoothly in the ring to give the judges the most advantageous view of the client's dog as possible. A skilled handler make a dog come across as the best among equals. Many a dog owes the letter "Ch." (Champion) before its name to the person on the business end of the leash.

Handling is a learn-by-doing job, almost invariably an outgrowth of earlier skills in obedience training and grooming. Professional handlers view themselves as creative people, able to transform, even inspire, an ungainly animal to become an almost charismatic work of art by the steps they take before the show and the moves they make in the ring. They pride themselves on the pay-off that comes from infinite attention to detail.

There is also a large and lucrative opportunity for field dog trainers. These dogs must be so skilled and accomplished that the training is almost always done by a professional.

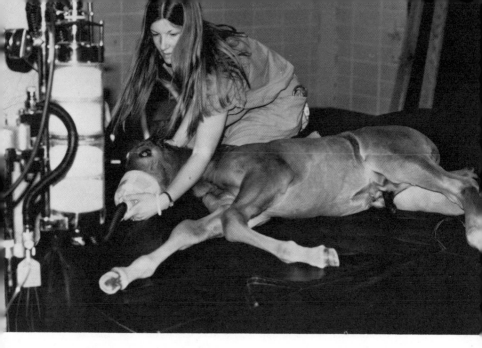

Horses require various kinds of attention, including surgery (upper) and shoeing (lower). Photos: University of Illinois College of Veterinary Medicine.

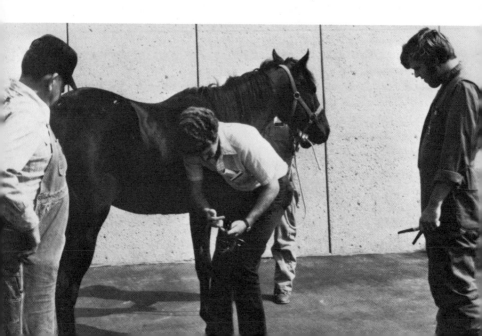

CHAPTER 14

CAREERS WITH HORSES

A nonfatal but very pronounced affliction strikes many youngsters from 8 to 12 and often lasts to the late teen years, or for life. It's name: "horse fever." If you have it, you know all the symptoms—and you probably enjoy every one!

Whether the ailment can, or should, form the basis of a career with horses is another matter, one that particularly has to do with money. Unless you have a good bit of it, or are willing to work long and hard for very little of it, you may be better off riding horses than raising them or otherwise involving yourself with them financially.

Yet for the apt and dedicated victim of horse fever, there are many career opportunities. Keep in mind (as we mentioned with dog careers) that success may well depend on having a variety of talents. Your chances for eventual financial success are better if you generalize rather than specialize. This rule can, of course, be broken by the truly skilled specialist. But please keep the concept of combining your talents in mind as you read about these separate horse careers.

HORSE BREEDER

It is appropriate to begin equine careers with the one specialty that makes all the others possible. Although fossils from millions of years ago show that America once had horses, there were none when Columbus arrived. The Spanish explorers DeSoto and Coronado brought the first horses to this country. The wild horses of the American West are believed to have descended from them, or from those brought to our shores by 17th Century Spanish missionaries. The Colonists brought horses, too, and it was then that breeding became a career. Today's horse breeder is a "descendant" of sorts from—among other famous Americans—George Washington.

Horse breeding generally calls for more formal education and money than most other equine careers. The breeder needs to know the nature and characteristics of the horses being bred—and there are many distinct breeds within the classifications of pony, light horse and draft horse. The breeder must have a working knowledge of: nutritious feeding practices; selection of stallions and mares for breeding (genetics); safe foaling (birthing); healthy stabling conditions; horse exercise needs; equine diseases and first aid; safe horse transportation; good record-keeping and sound business practices; marketing knowledge—where and how to advertise, proper pricing, good salesmanship.

These are the things that protect the breeder's profit. Considering the hefty investment needed in horses, pastureland, buildings, feeds, employees, vans and veterinary fees, making a profit calls for careful attention to every detail.

For every famous racing stable with its outstanding winners, there are scores of others that do not make a profit, so chancy is Thoroughbred racing. Many successful horse breeders prefer to pass up the high-rolling in favor of breeding sound, saleable ponies and light (pleasure) horses which are honestly represented and sold at fair prices. Understandably, many horse breeders not only breed and raise horses for sale, but offer the other services such as boarding and riding instruction covered in this chapter, to make their considerable investment pay on a daily basis.

How does the horse breeder learn to evaluate mares and stallions as producers of quality foals? Experience as a horse farm employee is the best way for you to start, but formal education in high school and beyond, at a land grant or agricultural college is recommended. High school and college courses should include animal husbandry, animal science, biology, business management, economics, farm management, genetics and the basics of animal health and veterinary medicine. College tuition can cost from $3,000 to $8,000 or more a year, depending on whether or not you must go out-of-state for your college.

From a start in agricultural or vo-tech high school and membership in a 4-H Club or Future Farmers of America chapter, you could work on a horse farm during summers and between semesters at college. Considering the relatively low pay, it may take time to save enough to buy your first mare to breed or stallion to place at stud, but that should be your goal.

With all the variables of expense versus income, it is hard to say what a horse breeder can earn from her or his entrepreneurial business...but the better the breeding involved, the higher the price of the product. The hours of outdoor work are long, the challenges are considerable. They are offset by having the breeding farm as your country home, and by the daily joy of living, working with, and developing your own horses.

STABLE OWNER AND RIDING INSTRUCTOR

Kate Goldenberg, a Bedminster, Pennsylvania, riding instructor and stable owner, feels that most self-owned animal businesses are expensive propositions. "In my work, fencing, grain, safety features on stalls—all these cost money. And if you don't have quality, people won't board with you. They have to trust you to care for their animals."

As riding instructor, trainer, breeder and horse farm manager with her husband Kenny, Kate Goldenberg is aware of this faith placed in her. For her, animal care is a full-time job that cuts no corners. Make that a 24-hour job—mares have a tendency to foal at night!

Kate also sees her field in terms of intrinsic rewards. "There may be a satisfaction in getting rich," she says, "but if you look out over your beautiful farm and animals and don't have a penny in your pocket, you are rich." Like many professionals, Kate cautions: "Don't confuse an affection for horses with an aptitude for working with them. Do stable work, either as a volunteer or for a little pay, to make sure you're up to the demands that animals make—they can be confining."

Like most people who operate riding facilities for profit, Kate Goldenberg offers a variety of services, from boarding others' horses to giving lessons and leading trail rides with her own animals—even staging horse shows on her farm.

Here, reprinted by permission, is a list of countryside stables north of Philadelphia, Pennsylvania. It appeared in "The Chestnut Hill Local," a weekly newspaper. It is typical of the services offered and the prices charged by stable operators.

While a good indicator of prices, no list such as this can cover the costs of operating a riding business. Those who do it for a living agree on one thing: do it right, or not at all. A damp, drafty stable, an over-age horse van, and inadequate cleaning, feeding, exercise and grooming will cost more in equine ill-health and other problems than such short-cutting will save.

Volunteering is the best way to get your feet muddy (if not wet) in the horse world. Working with an experienced stable operator, you'll learn how to ride for pleasure and for show, how to groom, saddle and feed horses, how to treat simple ailments that do not need a veterinarian's attention—and how to recognize troubles that do. As a start, you may muck out the horses' stalls, that never-ending job that gave Hercules fits at the Aegean stables! But mucking, like every other chore, goes with the territory.

One very worthwhile task for the volunteer and the dedicated stable owner is giving riding lessons to the handicapped, also called therapeutic riding. Although the idea is relatively new, it is growing in popularity. Most participating organizations are members of NARHA, the North American Riding for the Handicapped Association. NARHA supervises therapeutic riding programs to see that their safety standards and teaching methods are followed. Only gentle, specially-schooled horses and ponies are used, and instruction is given by highly-qualified professionals. Therapeutic riding helps physically handicapped, mentally retarded, learning-disabled and emotionally disturbed children and adults adjust to and improve their handicapping conditions. It improves coordination, posture, balance, strength and muscle tone. It also fosters feelings of self-worth, self-confidence, and accomplishment.

Where would you fit in to such a program? Probably as a volunteer *walker* who would move alongside the horse or pony, helping the handicapped rider stay balanced, comfortable, at ease and in control. You could do this independently with a participating stable, or—more usually—as a member of a Scout or 4-H group.

As part of your learning experience as a stable hand, you could perform similar duties with a riding instructor as he or she conducts beginners' lessons for normal students. It's a good beginning in learning to be a full-fledged riding instructor.

A riding instructor must be able to do two things well: to ride proficiently, and to convey that skill to others. The first attribute is self-evident; only the person capable of managing any horse in any situation from trail riding to show jumping with the confidence built through experience can do a proper job of teaching.

Communicating your skills calls for the ability to recognize and correct their lack in your students. Almost anyone can ride—badly. But achieving a proper seat and maintaining control through the use of hand and leg "aids" that a horse knows and will respond to are skills that must be taught. When beginning riders are instinctively good, the instructor must be able to recognize these skills and teach the rider how to improve on them. With most beginners, the instructor must be able to correct a host of mistakes and improve the student's performance by word and by example. With some students, this requires almost infinite patience.

The self-employed riding instructor charges from $8 to $20 for a riding lesson, depending on the number of students (the private lesson is more expensive) and the nature of the lesson. (For dressage or advanced jumping, the price may be as fancy as the hoofwork.) These prices are estimates, per-hour.

HORSE TRAINER

Although there are certain procedures common to all forms of horse training, there are as many variations as there are needs for horses (cowponies are trained with different techniques than jumpers, for instance).

Among the traits shared by all horse trainers are excellent physical condition, an understanding of horse psychology and health, patience, gentleness, and the willingness to work long hours for relatively little pay.

The sooner a trainer can work with a colt, the better. It's not unusual for a trainer to work for short periods with a foal, building a relationship through petting, soothing words and gentle handling. The growing animal is taught in successive stages over a year or longer to accept a halter and be led on a short line without fear. The line is gradually lengthened and the colt is taught to start and stop on command, to go through its gaits (walk, trot, canter, perhaps pace, singlefoot or run, depending on breed and training). It is taught to stand still for grooming and to accept the confines of stableyard, barn and ring. Later, it learns to accept bit, bridle, saddle and harness cart, not always in this order. Eventually comes riding, sometimes by the familiar trainer, often by a co-trainer or assistant who rides while the trainer directs the proceedings, with—and later without—the long line. With consistency and kindness, the rider-trainer schools the young horse in the meaning of commands given by reins, knees and heels. These aids are used to teach the horse when to change gait, to slow, turn and stop, so that the response will be the same no matter who is riding.

Training uses the punishment-reward system, not with treats but with gentle words, pats and relaxation in the saddle for a good performance; more stern speech, leg and rein pressure to say in essence, "Not so hot—let's try that again." Stronger punishment is used sparingly and with great discretion.

That's basic training. Horses can be trained more specifically, depending on breed and purpose, and many trainers specialize. A hunter or show horse is taught to jump; a cowpony to change gait, stop, and turn instantly and accurately, and to react to the pull of the roped steer; a harness racer to trot or pace at speed; dressage and circus horses are patiently trained for their special work.

Horse trainers, specialized or not, learn their art by doing—usually starting as apprentices to established trainers. On a dude ranch or at a riding academy, you may begin as a groom and advance to trail ride leader and riding instructor. At racing stables and tracks, dedicated youngsters often begin as grooms, exercise riders and hotwalkers who walk horses to exercise them and to cool them down after races or practice runs. This work develops the students' own riding talents.

Training, like instructing, is not known for high pay. The "plus" side for you may be the chance to learn on the job, to work largely outdoors, to work seasonally or full-time, and—with luck and talent—to make a living based largely on your own increasing abilities rather than on formal education beyond high school (more on this later).

The big money-makers among horse trainers are those able to recognize and develop equine and human talent for showmanship and particularly for racing. The race horse trainer rarely owns the horses he or she trains, but trains them for the owners of stud farms and racing stables. The trainer's skills extend to selecting the best of the horses in his or her charge for specific events, and picking the right rider as well. In the case of show horses, the rider may be the owner, and the trainer may work with rider and mount as a team.

The more experienced race horse trainers are often paid a percentage of their horses' winnings—usually 10%—and this may result in earnings of $100,000 or more a year. More down-to-earth is the $400 a month a novice trainer may earn, or the approximately $10,000 annual income which is the average for the profession.

PROFESSIONAL RIDERS

Anyone who primarily earns a living by riding horses is technically a professional rider. But the term also applies to Grand Prix horse show contestants, and is usually reserved for harness racing drivers and flat racing jockeys. They are professionals inasmuch as they are paid in proportion to their skills and victories versus defeats, just as other professional athletes are. Being a Grand Prix rider, harness driver or jockey generally isn't something a "horse person" starts off being; rather, it is something they eventually may become after months or years of long hours spent in hard, time-consuming work with horses.

Talent and luck have a lot to do with whether or not you as an exerciser or apprentice trainer ever get a shot at professional riding. Size and weight aren't all-important in Grand Prix, competitive dressage, circus work or even in harness racing, but to the would-be Thoroughbred jockey, less is more. A normal weight without constant dieting of 105 to 112 pounds is essential; the less weight a race horse carries, the better.

Alison Kramer of New Jersey is 22 years old. She fell in love with horses at age 11 when she learned to ride at an equestrian school. After graduating from high school, Alison worked with show horses and later had a job training yearlings.

For the last five years, Alison has worked as an exercise girl at race tracks in New Jersey, New York, and Florida, "but I always wanted to be a jockey," she says.

Finally, in May, 1983, trainer Henry Carroll let her race "Quick Hitch" at Monmouth (NJ) Race Course. Although she finished sixth in a ten-horse race, "it was a great experience."

For every Steve Cauthen—the first jockey to earn $6,000,000 for riding 488 winners in one year—there are hundreds who work under contract to racing stable owners for a salary-plus-bonus for wins, or who freelance, picking up "rides" at the request of trainers who match them with suitable horses. Travel expenses and costly riding gear are usually the jockey's responsibility, and their costs can cut severely into earnings— jockeys must travel to race "meetings" throughout the country. Even at that, incomes of $50,000 and more a year are not unusual for jockeys with good reputations—but not celebrity status. Racing is held only when, and where, it is warm but not hot. In this seasonal work, there may be several "dry" months a year—and jockeying is definitely an early-retirement career. Retired jockeys often work in other areas of racing. One English steeplechaser Dick Francis, has become a highly successful mystery novel writer!

OTHER TRACK CAREERS—AND BLACKSMITHING

There are careers on race tracks for experienced people who work with horses but don't necessarily ride them. During a meeting, race tracks will employ racing secretaries, stewards, judges, veterinarians, specialists who tattoo horses' lips to identify them, and identifiers who verify the horses' identities against their tattoos and their registration papers before they can race.

Then, there is the blacksmith, often called a smith, farrier, or horse shoer. Only the most skilled may be licensed to work at race tracks, but whether at the track or the horse farm, the job is equally demanding.

We'll bet there's at least one blacksmith whose truck reads "We Make Horse Calls," for indeed they do. The "village smithy" no longer stands "under the spreading chestnut tree" but rolls instead, from stud farm to race track to riding academy. Although there are some women farriers, Longfellow's poetic line, "The smith a mighty man is he" generally holds true, for horse shoeing calls for a strong back, legs, and arms. It's work that should be started early in life, according to professionals.

There is a difference, though. Today's blacksmith is more equine podiatrist than ironworker. In fact, with most race horses, the shoe of choice is lightweight aluminum. In many cases, the inbreeding that has been used to develop race horses with great speed may also have created the hoof problems which the blacksmith must recognize and correct. This is done by tailoring the fit of the shoe. Although the farrier's experience helps determine the correction that must be made, the desired result is often a matter of trying and trying again until the race horse's speed, gait, and comfort are right.

The blacksmith's day starts early—especially at race tracks. Each previous day's thrown shoes or other problems must be solved before the horses' morning workouts. The rest of the day at the races is taken up with routine shoe changes and consulting with trainers and jockeys on problems that arise.

Race track work usually involves testing and licensing, but whether or not a farrier works at the track, he or she may take smithing courses in vo-tech high school as career preparation, and definitely should serve an apprenticeship with a skilled smith. A blacksmith must, of course, be able to handle horses, often when they are not on their best behavior. Need for tailoring and special shoes extends to show and pleasure horses, too.

In addition to a sturdy pickup truck, 4 x 4 or van, today's blacksmith needs to invest in the equipment of the craft: powered grinder, drill press, forge, anvil, gas torches and finishing tools (knives, rasps, etc.). This is a several-thousand-dollar investment.

A foot trim may be $9 to $12, a set of shoes, $30 or more. An experienced blacksmith may be able to shoe from 5 to 10 horses a day, depending on the travel involved. The money is such that a capable blacksmith with a following can be assured of a good living plus a fair degree of independence.

EDUCATION

The education in high school and beyond described in the horse breeder profile would be excellent training for most horse careers, as a supplement to learning-by-doing. There are a small but growing number of colleges and junior colleges that offer courses related to horsemanship. Some schools of equitation offer certificates of proficiency. The Central Kentucky Vocational-Technical School in Lexington offers a 40-week classroom, horse farm and race track course that prepares students for jobs as racetrack officials.

Harcum Junior College in Bryn Mawr, Pennsylvania, is close to the world-famous Devon Horse Show grounds; Chesterland, the site of national horse trials; and the Radnor Hunt Club. Over the past ten years, Harcum has established itself in the field of animal health care by offering majors in many animal care areas. The school has recently added an Associate Degree program in Equine Studies. Among the electives: equine breeding; therapeutic riding; equine business management; teaching of equitation. To prepare for these careers, students at Harcum take courses in animal biology, equine health and disease, lameness, equitation theory, equitation instruction, organization of events, stable management and equine business management.

The Harcum program may well have its equivalent in other parts of the country. Among other colleges offering equine programs are Smith and Centenary. The Potomac Horse Center near Washington, DC offers a Horsemaster's Certificate, and the Los Alamos (NM) Dressage Center offers a Certificate of Training in this riding specialty.

IN CLOSING...

We hope this book has helped you to learn about today's many animal career opportunities, and to choose the one that best suits your aspirations and abilities.

No matter which career you select, you can take pride in respecting and working with animals. In doing so, you will continue a relationship as old as civilization itself—but for you, it will be only The Beginning.

APPENDIX A

PROGRAMS IN ANIMAL TECHNOLOGY

ALABAMA
Snead State Junior College
Animal Hospital Technology
 Program
Boaz, AL 35957
205/593-5120

CALIFORNIA
Cosumnes River College
Animal Health Technology
 Program
8401 Center Parkway
Sacramento, CA 95823
916/689-1000

Hartnell College
Animal Health Technician
 Program
156 Homestead Avenue
Salinas, CA 93901
408/758-8211

Los Angeles Pierce College
Animal Health Technology
 Program
6201 Winnetka Avenue
Woodland Hills, CA 92101
213/347-0551

Mt. San Antonio College
Animal Health Technology
 Program
1100 North Grand Avenue
Walnut, CA 91789
714/594-5611

Orange Coast College
Animal Health Technology
 Program
2701 Fairview Road
Costa Mesa, CA 92626
714/556-5982

San Diego Mesa College
Animal Health Technology
 Program
7250 Mesa College Drive
San Diego, CA 92111
619/230-6811

Yuba College
Animal Health Technician
 Program
Beale Road and Linda Avenue
Marysville, CA 95901
916/742-7351

COLORADO
Colorado Mountain College
Animal Health Technology
 Program
West Campus
Glenwood Springs, CO 81601
303/945-7481

Bel-Rea Institute of
 Animal Technology
9870 East Alameda
Denver, CO 80231
303-366-2639

CONNECTICUT
Quinnipiac College
Laboratory Animal Technology
Mt. Carmel Avenue
Hamden, CT 06518
203/288-5251

FLORIDA
St. Petersburg Junior College
Veterinary Technology Program
Box 13489
St. Petersburg, FL 33833
813/381-0681

GEORGIA
Abraham Baldwin Agricultural
 College
Veterinary Technology Program
Box 8, ABAC Station
Tifton, GA 31793
912/386-3547

Fort Valley State College
Veterinary Technology Program
Fort Valley, CA 31030
912/825-6353

ILLINOIS
Parkland College
Veterinary Technology Program
2400 Bradley
Champaign, IL 61820
217/351-2394

INDIANA
Purdue University
School of Veterinary Medicine
Veterinary Technology Program
West Lafayette, IN 47907
317/494-7619

KANSAS
Colby Community College
Animal Technology Program
1255 South Range
Colby, KS 67701
913/462-3985

KENTUCKY
Morehead State University
Veterinary Technology Program
Box 72
Morehead, KY 40351
606/783-2025

LOUISIANA
Northwestern State University
 of Louisiana
Veterinary Technology Program
Dept. of Agricultural Sciences
Natchitoches, LA 71457
318/357-5912

MAINE
University of Maine
Animal Medical Technology
 Program
Dept. of Animal &
 Veterinary Sciences
Orono, ME 04473
207/581-1110

MARYLAND
Essex Community College
Animal Science Technology
 Program
7201 Rossville Blvd.
Baltimore, MD 21237
301/682-6000

Garrett Community College
Veterinary Technology Program
McHenry, MD 21541
301/387-6666

MASSACHUSETTS
Newbury Junior College
Animal Health Technician
  Program
921 Boylston Street
Boston, MA 02115
617/429-6810
(Holliston Campus)

Becker Junior College
Veterinary Assistant Program
1003 Old Main Street
Leicester, MA 01524
617/892-8122

MICHIGAN
Macomb County College
Veterinary Technician Program
Center Campus
44575 Garfield Road
Mt. Clemens, MI 48044
313/286-2169

Michigan State University
College of Veterinary Medicine
Animal Technology Program
East Lansing, MI 48823
517/353-7267

Wayne County Community
  College
Veterinary Technician
  Training Program
540 E. Canfield
Detroit, MI 48201
313/577-1156

MINNESOTA
Medical Institute of Minnesota
Veterinary Technician Program
2309 Nicollet Avenue
Minneapolis, MN 55404
612/871-8481

University of Minnesota
Animal Health Technology
  Program
Waseca, MN 56093
507/835-1000

MISSOURI
Maple Woods Community
  College
Animal Health Technology
  Program
2601 N.W. Barry Road
Kansas City, MO 64156
816/436-6500

Northeast Missouri
  State University
Animal Health Technology
  Program
Kirksville, MO 63501
816/785-4574

Jefferson College
Animal Health Technology
  Program
Hillsboro, MO 63050
314/789-3951

NEBRASKA
University of Nebraska
School of Technical Agriculture
Veterinary Technology Program
Curtis, NE 69025
308/367-4124

NEW JERSEY
Camden County College
Animal Science Technology
  Program
P.O. Box 200
Blackwood, NJ 08012
609/227-7200

NEW YORK
La Guardia Community College
The City University
of New York
Animal Health Technology
Program
21-10 Thomson Avenue
Long Island City, NY 11101
212/626-5077

State University of New York
Agricultural & Technical
College
Veterinary Science Technology
Program
Delhi, NY 13753
607/746-4262

State University of New York
Agricultural & Technical
College
Agriculture & Life Sciences
Veterinary Science Technology
Program
Canton, NY 13617
315/386-7011-7410

NORTH CAROLINA
Central Carolina Technical
Institute
Veterinary Medical Technology
Program
1105 Kelly Drive
Sanford, NC 27330
919/775-5401

NORTH DAKOTA
North Dakota State University
Animal Health Technician
Program
Dept. of Veterinary Science
Fargo, ND 58102
701/237-7511

OHIO
Columbus Technical Institute
Animal Health Technology
Program
550 East Springs Street
Columbus, OH 43215
614/227-2512

Raymond Walters College
Animal Health Technology
Program
University of Cincinnati
Cincinnati, OH 45221
513/872/5171

OKLAHOMA
Murray State College
Veterinary Assistant Technology
Program
Tisbomingo, OK 73460
405/371/2371

PENNSYLVANIA
Harcum Junior College
Animal Technician Program
Bryn Mawr, PA 19010
215/525-4100

Median School of Allied
  Health Careers
Animal Health Technology
  Program
121 - 9th Street
Pittsburgh, PA 15222
412/391-7021

SOUTH CAROLINA
Tri-County Technical College
Animal Health Technology
  Program
P.O. Box 587
Pendleton, SC 29670
803/646-3227

SOUTH DAKOTA
National College
Animal Health Care Program
P.O. Box 302
Rapid City, SD 57709
800/843-8892

TENNESSEE
Columbia State
  Community College
Animal Health Technology
  Program
Columbia, TN 38401
615/388-0120

TEXAS
Cedar Valley College
Animal Medical Technology
  Program
3030 N. Dallas Avenue
Lancaster, TX 75134

Sul Ross State University
Range Animal Science Dept.
Animal Health Technology

Program
Alpine, TX 79830
915/837-8205

Texas State Technical Institute
Animal Medical Technology
  Program
James Connally Campus
Waco, TX 76705
817/799-3611

UTAH
Brigham Young University
Animal Health Technology
  Program
Provo, UT 84602
801/378-4294

VIRGINIA
Blue Ridge Community College
Animal Technology Program
Box 80
Weyers Cave, VA 24486
703/234-9261

Northern Virginia Community
  College
Animal Science Technology
  Program
Loudoun Campus
1000 Harry Flood Byrd Hwy.
Sterling, VA 22170
703/323-4501

WASHINGTON
Fort Steilacoom Community
  College
Animal Technology Program
9401 Farwest Dr., S.W.
Tacoma, WA 98498
206/964-6665

WEST VIRGINIA
Fairmont State College
Veterinary Assistant Technology
  Program
Fairmont, WV 26554
304/367-4268

WISCONSIN
Madison Area Technical
  College
Animal Technician Program
211 North Carroll Street
Madison, WI 53703
608/266-5001

WYOMING
Eastern Wyoming College
Animal Health Technology
  Program
3200 West C. Street
Torrington, WY 82240
307/532-7111

APPENDIX B

RELATED READING

Pamphlets

Animal Hospital Attendants and Animal Technicians (Occupational Brief 480). Chronicle Guidance Publications, Inc., P.O. Box 271, Moravia, NY 13118.

Animal Technology. American Veterinary Medical Association, 930 North Meacham Road, Schaumburg, IL 60196.

Careers in Zoo Keeping. Brookfield Zoo Chapter, American Association of Zoo Keepers, Chicago Zoological Society, Brookfield Zoo, Brookfield, IL 60513.

Today's Veterinarian. American Veterinary Medical Association, 930 Meacham Road, Schaumburg, IL 60196.

Veterinarians (Occupational Brief 83). Chronicle Guidance Publications, Inc., P.O. Box 271, Moravia, NY 13118.

A Wildlife Conservation Career For You. The Wildlife Society, Suite 611, 7101 Wisconsin Avenue, Washington, DC 20014.

*Zoo and Aquarium Careers.*The American Association of Zoological Parks and Aquariums, Oglebay Park, Wheeling, WV 26003.

Zoo Jobs. Office of Education–Information, National Zoological Park, Washington, DC 20009.

Books

Animal Doctors: What It's Like to be a Veterinarian and How to Become One, by Patricia Curtis. 1977. Delacorte Press, 1 Dag Hammarskjold Plaza, New York, NY 10017.

Ms. Veterinarian, by Mary Price Lee. 1976. Westminster Press, Witherspoon Building, Philadelphia, PA 19101.

Opportunities in Biological Sciences, by Charles Winter. 1984. National Textbook Company, 4255 West Touhy Avenue, Lincolnwood, IL 60646.

Your Future in Veterinary Medicine, by Wayne H. Riser, D.V.M. 1976. Arco Publishing Company, 219 Park Avenue South, New York, NY 10003.

Zoo Careers, by William Bridges. 1971. William Morrow and Company, 105 Madison Avenue, New York, NY 10016.